THE UNI
THE COLLEGE OF RIPON
AND YORK ST. JOHN
SU

1994

95

54673

WITHDRAWN 16/3/24

MORE TALK OF ALEXANDER

NOTE

Text references to photographs are given with the term "plate" followed by a number to be found in the inset between pages 32 and 33. Text references to drawings and diagrams are given with the term "figure" or "Fig.".

Contents

INTRODUCTION

THE LAST FEW years have seen a tremendous upsurge of interest in the work of Matthias Alexander. I would like to think that some of this has been due to my book *The Alexander Principle*, but it seems more likely that the time had become right, and that my book simply served as a catalyst. A great deal had already been written about Alexander and his own four books had always had a devoted following: but we have to remember that his own books were written in the first half of the twentieth century, well before the modern explosion of knowledge in the fields of education, medicine, biology and psychology. He was not only treading new ground—he had to use old words in new ways without the modern terminology which now makes explanation so much easier.

Inevitably much of what was first written about Alexander now seems to have a period flavour. Indeed it is with slight embarrassment that I include some of my own earlier writings—the broad argument, the sweeping conclusions, the quotations from a limited number of sources. But the fact is that there is suddenly a huge new public for Alexander's ideas, and this new public wants to know much more about our origins and experimentations. Many of them want to know how it could have been that these exciting new ideas did not catch on before. Those of us who have tried to be midwives to Alexander's work can only reply that we did our best, but that in what can now be seen to have been an over-rigid and restricted society, those in authority did not want to hear about approaches which ran counter to their established ways.

Not only this. Alexander was a maverick, an eccentric who did not disguise the distaste which he felt for inadequate educational and medical procedures. His manner was characterized by a directness and forthright intolerance which might delight the intelligent non-academic, but which infuriated those who found themselves at the receiving end.

I first started collecting together some of the earliest writings on Alexander in 1945, and I published a small booklet of these under a title which T. S. Eliot suggested to me, *Knowing How to Stop*. It proved suprisingly popular as an introduction to Alexander's work and encouraged by its success I began to collect together further material. The best of this material was published in the *Alexander Journal* and this was circulated amongst Alexander teachers and amongst their pupils and patients. It never reached a very large public and expense has made it difficult to produce on a regular basis.

Many of these earlier articles, although excellent on their own, were saying much the same thing in only a slightly different way, and I have therefore left out of this present book those whose contents are covered elsewhere. For many reasons I have also had to leave out excellent articles on the application of Alexander's work to industry, criminology, and mountaineering, but I have been extremely fortunate in being allowed to publish the Nobel Oration which Professor Nikolaas Tinbergen delivered when he was given the Nobel Prize in Medicine in 1973. It might be said that Alexander's work really came of age at this point, when it was made the central feature of the Nobel Prize Oration.

There are also many other new papers which have not yet appeared in print, including Professor Tinbergen's Memorial Lecture at the Royal Society of Medicine; and I have included some papers of my own which have been printed in specialized medical journals and which are not easily available.

The material has not been easy to classify, but there is a clear distinction between those who are writing to give their personal reactions to what Alexander did and taught, and those who are attempting to comment upon the relationship of his work to other fields of study. Much of the writing contains both of these aspects, but it seems to me helpful to divide up the material into (1) Descriptions, (2) Applications, and (3) Objections.

After a good deal of deliberation, I have included the *Lancet*'s summary of the successful legal action which Alexander brought against the South African government. Historians will, I think, find the voluminous evidence given in this trial a goldmine of information, not only because of the nonsense which was talked about Alexander, but also because of the almost hysterical reactions of some eminent members of the medical profession in this country and in South Africa. I have also included most of our leading counsel's opening address since it is an excellent summary of some of Alexander's work. Alexander had brought his action against the South African government at a time—just post-Smuts—when their methods were not so generally disliked as they are at present. Observers of the South African scene will be intrigued to see that the notorious Oswald Pirow was the defending counsel for that government, and that Alexander's second counsel was Bram Fischer, who was subsequently to be imprisoned by the South African government and died in jail—I count myself fortunate in having got to know this delightful and humane man, and indeed the others of a liberal viewpoint who helped us. Since Alexander was old and not strong enough to appear,

I had the gruelling, but, in retrospect, exciting experience of spending two days in cross-examination by Pirow on some of Alexander's less defensible ideas.

Alexander's work has developed recently into two distinct streams. There has always been an unorthodox "fringe" surrounding his work, and rather surprisingly this now shows itself in the educational rather than in the medical field. Various forms of esoteric movement-training and "body-contact" disciplines have seemed to some people to have close affinities with Alexander's work, although it should be pointed out that it was only as a result of medical and scientific work that the technique has managed to become established in Colleges of Further Education—notably in music, drama, and speech-training colleges. Because of its "fringe" educational proponents, it cannot be said to have made any appreciable impact on the normal school and university educational curriculum. Indeed, in any case, the personal one-to-one relationship which Alexander's work involves will always be more suited to the one-to-one setting which medical work involves, rather than to the group approach of most school and university education. Inevitably those who have tried to use Alexander's work in an educational field have found it difficult to resist the demand for such group work: and once this demand is acceded to, essential Alexander detail has usually been lost, although it can only be a question of time before someone dedicated to the scientific approach will make the necessary educational breakthrough.

The present time is an exciting and important one for the development of Alexander's work. A good test of any man's importance is his endurance in the public mind after his death. The extent of his impact in his lifetime may not be as significant as the later persistence and spread of what he stood for. Many headliners pass into oblivion after their death.

Matthias Alexander was not fashionable in his lifetime. A very few people thought he was saying something crucially important and those of us who hung on and supported him have sometimes been accused of exaggerated enthusiasm. We might reply that when you have to whistle to keep your spirits up, the whistle is bound to seem a little shrill at times. If there is sometimes a shrill note in some of the papers in this book, there is also a stream of good commonsense. I appreciate only too well that the statistical background which doctors and scientists will eventually need is not very much in evidence: but since research funds have simply not been forthcoming to help us, reports have had to be, in the main, observational and descriptive: the clinical virtues. It is my hope that the wide range of topics which are touched on here will lead a next generation of teachers and researchers to extend their work into the various fields touched on here, as well as into many others.

Chapters 2, 4, 5, 6, 7, 11, 12, 13, 14, 15, 16, 23, 24, 26, 28, 31 and 35 are reprinted from the *Alexander Journal* of which I am the editor. Part 2 of chapter 8, "An Investigation into Kinaesthesia", was published by permission of the Army Council and formerly appeared in the *Medical Press and Circular*; whilst part 3 of the same chapter, "Postural Deformity", is reprinted by permission of the Royal Society of Medicine, to which it was delivered as part of a symposium on postural deformity. Chapters 10 and 22 are reprinted by permission of the *British Journal of Physical Medicine*. The extract from *The Study of Instinct* by Professor N. Tinbergen reprinted in chapter 29 is done so with permission of the Oxford University Press; whilst his Nobel Oration, chapter 30, is reprinted with the permission of the Nobel Foundation.

I am grateful to Douglas Newton for help with my article on Visual Art, chapter 19; and I should, above all, like to express my thanks to my wife, Marjory, for her constant help in preparing this material, and to the teachers of the Alexander Institute who have given such helpful advice and criticism: in particular to those who helped so much in the difficult early years—Joyce Wodeman, Muriel Maconochie, Dick Walker and Inge Henderson.

DESCRIPTIONS

ONE

The Teaching of F. Matthias Alexander
by Marjory Alexander Barlow

(An Alexander Memorial Lecture given in November 1965)

THESE ANNUAL LECTURES were instituted as a memorial to F. M. Alexander. A decade has passed since his death on 10 October 1955 so this is perhaps an appropriate moment to pass in review the knowledge which he left us, and to recall aspects of his teaching which may be in danger of being forgotten and ultimately lost, as the psychophysical benefits of his work become better known. An institution, said Emerson, is the lengthened shadow of one man—we, in this Society, are the rapidly lengthening shadow of Alexander. This lecture is a plea that as the shadow grows we may take care not to lose the substance.

It must be remembered that in order to discuss or analyse anything the nature of language forces us to speak in a separative way. The living human being is a whole—works well or badly as a whole—and living experiences are integrated and simultaneous in a way which cannot be expressed in words. Physical and mental aspects of any activity are in fact one, but have to be separated for purposes of discussion.

The idea that posture affects well-being is a very ancient one. We know that the Greeks were concerned with it, that Victorian young ladies used backboards to encourage straight spines, and that posture training in the gymnasium is part of the accepted curriculum in schools. Many eastern religions and disciplines contained instructions about the carriage and comportment of the body.

We might almost speak of the noble lineage of this idea, since so many of the expressions enshrined in our language indicate a knowledge that bodily attitude betrays inner states of mind or dominant characteristics. We speak of "a spineless creature", "having no backbone", "losing our heads" or "being level-headed"—we all know what it is to be "beside ourselves". The Bible abounds in references to a stiff-necked generation—"The stiff-necked and the unbelievers shall be punished" and "they stiffened their necks that they might not hear the word of the Lord" are two nice ones.

During the last 30 years, at least, the importance of body-mechanics has been widely recognized. Alexander found that the problem of posture was a much more fundamental one than had been suspected. He did not use the word posture, because it was too limited a concept for the nature of the discoveries he had made, which showed that bad "posture" or, as he preferred to call it, "misuse of the self" was the end result of much deeper wrong processes, involving the whole person. In fact, of bad habits "woven in the weakness of the changing body", as Eliot puts it.

One of the things he meant by the "use of the self" was the way in which the various parts of the body are related to one another in actually living, moving and having our being.

Posture implies fixed positions, and right and wrong ways of sitting, standing, etc., and posture training is based on the inadequate assumption that bad posture can be altered satisfactorily from the *outside*, by *doing* something different.

To start with the wrong end of the stick—because the wrong end is observable—Alexander found that we live in almost complete ignorance of the way we use the body—that most people are distorting the form, and impairing the working of the whole organism, by bad co-ordination, muscular overtension and misuse of the parts of the body in their relationship to one another.

The body is an instrument—it is the instrument through which we live—it can be capable of very fine and subtle perceptions. Professor A. N. Whitehead wrote in his book *The Romantic Reaction*, "The unity of the perceptual field, therefore, must be a unity of bodily experience. Your perception takes place where you are AND IS ENTIRELY DEPENDENT ON HOW YOUR BODY IS FUNCTIONING." This instrument is being damaged and distorted in ways largely unconsidered until Alexander began to teach. It is being rendered gross, heavy and incapable of sensitive behaviour, by overtension and the resultant internal noise to which it is subject. This lack of peace in the body makes almost impossible the condition known as "peace of mind".

The form this misuse takes follows the same general pattern in everyone.

Invariably, the muscles of the neck are overcontracted, causing loss of the free poise of the head on top of the spine. This leads to over-contraction of some muscles of the trunk, and lack of proper tone in the other supporting muscles of the body. This results in exaggeration of the natural curves of the spine, and harmful pressure on the individual vertebrae of the spinal column and on the joints, coupled with overwork and wrong relationship of the limbs to the trunk.

In short we get a state of affairs where the work of supporting the body is being wrongly distributed—the form of the body distorted—and important functions such as breathing, blood circulation and digestion are working inefficiently and under enormous strain.

Another way of putting it is that the wrong general principle on which the body is being used is that of contracting every part of it *into* the nearest joint, beginning with the contraction of the head towards the trunk.

It is as if each of us is trying to take up the least possible amount of room in the Universe.

This unconscious way of mismanagement of the self produces states of disease—dis-ability—dis-comfort and general ill-health which baffle the ordinary doctor, and for which there is no help other than a radical change in the manner in which the person is using himself.

Fortunately, during the past fifteen years in England, medical research and the publication of scientific papers in medical textbooks and journals have resulted in a great increase in the number of doctors and psychiatrists who turn to teachers of the Alexander Technique for help with patients who are suffering from the effects of bad use.

To understand the difference between usual methods of posture training—or postural correction—and Alexander's teaching we must look again at his own story, re-examine our origins, and see how he arrived at the knowledge which has made possible a completely new approach to the problem of how to manage ourselves in the least harmful way.

Alexander began with the concrete—he had little time for theories or for ideas which had no practical application.

He was forced to his search by a disability which was interfering with his work as an actor and reciter. The problem seemed to be a specific difficulty—that of recurring hoarseness of his voice—but it led him to discover that a small and apparently isolated weakness could not be overcome without recourse to the total change of his whole self. And that attempts to change at the outer visible level—the usual way of trying to correct faults—were completely unavailing.

Here then was Alexander, a successful reciter with a passion for Shakespeare and a firm determination to become a great Shakespearean actor. All his ambitions were falling to pieces because his voice was not standing up to the demands being made upon it.

He sought medical advice. After disappointing trials of the

remedies, which worked improvements only as long as he refrained from using his voice, he came to a realization which was the first stroke of genius in a long series. He understood that he might be causing the trouble himself—that he might be putting strain on the vocal organs in some way which was unknown to him. Looking back from where we stand now, this step in a new direction in thinking about his problem, stands out clearly as the key to all that was to follow and shows Alexander's capacity for original thought and also the awkward way he had of not accepting anything at its face value. Even as a small boy this quality was evident. It is said that he was a perfect nuisance at the Dame School he attended in Tasmania because he invariably questioned everything he was taught, and asked his teachers how they knew that the information they were giving him was so.

There is no means of knowing how many people with Alexander's voice trouble have given up their careers as speakers, actors or singers because they accepted unthinkingly that, if medical treatment failed, there could be no other solution to their difficulties.

Alexander had now taken responsibility upon himself for his trouble. In order to observe what he did when he used his voice he practised speaking in front of mirrors. By patiently watching what he was doing he found, at length, that three rather peculiar things happened every time he spoke. There was a tendency to pull the head back, depress the larynx, and suck in air through the mouth. With these interferences went a tendency to raise his chest and shorten his whole body.

After much experimentation he found that if he could prevent the pulling back of the head the other misuses did not occur.

This was the second major discovery—namely, that the interference with the free poise of the head brought interference with the best working of the rest of his body in its train.

The dominance of the head in the hierarchy of the body he later called the Primary Control partly because, in unravelling the muddle of misuse, it is the first factor to be dealt with, and conditions the forms of misuse in the rest of the body.

The Primary Control, in its full definition, is the relationship between the head, the neck and the back. It is the Primary Control of the use of the body whether the use is good or bad.

Having discovered what might be causing the voice difficulties, Alexander now set about trying to correct these faults in the most obvious way. He tried to DO the opposite. But the more he struggled to do the right thing the more entangled he became.

He found that he couldn't stop these wrong habits by *trying* to do so. At last he realized that he hadn't got to *DO* something different—but to *stop* doing what he was doing already.

This is the next important principle in his teaching which turns upside down all the accepted notions about correcting something that is wrong. Usually if something is wrong we think we must DO something to put it right.

The new principle is that if something is wrong, we must find out what it is and stop doing it. The only cure for banging one's head against a wall is to stop.

The understanding of this principle is cardinal in any attempt to change misuse, and highlights one of the basic differences between this teaching and any other method.

It also provides a useful explanation of the work on a certain level. It can be formulated like this in answer to questions about what we do. "We teach people to become aware of the unnecessary strain and overtension they make in everything they do, so that they need not continue to misuse themselves in this way."

In other words we are concerned with giving our pupils the knowledge of how to liberate themselves from the cage of overtension in which they are imprisoned. So that the free natural use of the body can emerge. Cyril Connolly wrote in *The Unquiet Grave*—"inside every fat man is a thin one trying to get out". We might alter it thus, "Inside every tense man is a free one not knowing how to get out".

We are not teaching people what to do right—but how to stop wrong DOING. It is impossible to DO an UNDOING.

But to return to Alexander in front of his mirrors. He had now reached a deadlock. He knew what was wrong, he knew he couldn't DO anything to put it right. He had exhausted all ways of trying to alter what was going on FROM THE OUTSIDE.

The next step was to begin the journey inwards to the central place in himself where the trouble really lay. Along the route came the recognition that he could not trust his sense of feeling—that is, the kinaesthetic sense of how much muscular tension he was using. He found that what he could see happening in the mirror did not correspond at all with what he *felt* was happening. Up to this time no one had questioned the reliability of this faulty guide which we all use in judging what is going on in the body—how much tension we are making—and also where any part of the body is in relation to other parts, and to the whole. The kinaesthetic sense works partly through the muscle-spindles in the muscles, as well as from receptors in the joints. Muscle-spindles are tiny mechanisms whose function is to convey information from muscles to the higher centres of the brain about the state of muscles and to receive information back from the brain as to what the muscles should do about it. However, if too much tension is being made in the muscle, there comes a certain point when this "feed-back" between brain and muscle is put out of action, and we can no longer feel what we are doing. This is the scientific explanation of what Alexander called "faulty sensory appreciation" and this is the real "nigger in the wood pile" of our ignorance of what we are doing with ourselves when we are wrong. It makes clear *why* ordinary methods of putting things right without taking wrong feeling into account are likely to fail.

Alexander could not change anything by *doing*. He could not trust his feeling. He then saw that he had underestimated the strength of habit. What he observed in the mirror was the *end-result* of disordered inner patterns lying deep in the nervous system. And that these inner patterns of impulses, conveyed through the nervous system to the muscles acting on the bony structure and joints of the body, were operative perpetually, whether he was moving, speaking or sitting still.

In fact these inner patterns *were* him—insofar as his body was the outer manifestation of them.

The next step in the journey was taken when Alexander realized that the only place where he could begin to control the wrong habitual patterns was at the moment when the idea came to him to speak or move.

The moment when, whatever state of misuse he was in, it would be made worse as he went into action.

He had reached the only place, and the only moment in time, where change could begin, or where he could have any control over the habitual patterns of misuse, which were dominating everything he attempted to do.

This place, or this moment in time, was the instant that a stimulus to activity reached his consciousness. In the ordinary way, when a stimulus comes, we react to it in the only manner possible. The response is made without thought—without any knowledge on our part of what we are putting into motion. The reaction is the immediate response of the whole self, according to the habitual patterns of movement which we have developed from our earliest years. We have no choice in this, we can behave in no other way. We are bound in slavery to these unrecognized patterns just as surely as if we were automatons.

When Alexander reached understanding of this part of the problem he had found the key to all change. He understood at last in what way he must work.

We have now followed him in his journey from the outermost manifestation of misuse, that is the interference with the normal working of his whole body, resulting in the vocal failure, to the innermost point where he could stop this interference.

Let us now reverse the process and follow him on his way out again.

He had to make possible a pause or space between the stimulus and the response.

He decided to do this by saying "NO" to, or inhibiting, the immediate response. This proved to be the cornerstone on which all his later discoveries were made, and through which later changes were made possible. The word "inhibition" in this sense means the opposite of volition. Withholding consent to automatic reaction. It does *not* mean suppressing something in the sense in which it is used in psychoanalysis.

Having effectively prevented the old unconscious patterns from repeating themselves, and having made a break in the "perpetual motion" machine that he had become, Alexander then brought his brain into action by sending conscious, verbal instructions to the parts of the body which he had been unable to control before.

The first result of this way of working was to prevent the misuse of the head, neck and trunk. He had to be content for a time to give himself a stimulus, refuse to respond to it, and give the conscious messages or directions without actually carrying out a movement. This is the preparatory stage of what one might call "road building" or the "laying down of railway lines along which the train will eventually travel".

In time he was able to continue the new messages during movement.

Eventually the old wrong inner patterns were replaced by the new ones resulting in the co-ordinated, trouble-free working of his body.

In this way he put to a new use a faculty we all have and use in ordinary life. This faculty is intelligence, or the power of the brain to determine and direct what we wish to do. This power he now turned to the management and control of the use of his body, so that the whole of it became "informed with thought".

Let us now examine in detail the series of new orders or messages he was employing. The first and most important break in the old patterns came, as we have seen, when he said "NO" to the habitual reaction. He then ordered the muscles of the neck to release. The neck muscles are the only part of the body which can exert *direct* traction on the head, and it will be pulled back or down or sideways according to which group or groups of these muscles are being over-tensed.

No change in the poise of the head can happen while it is held in the grip of neck misuse. Moreover, the small sub-occipital muscles between the base of the skull and the top vertebrae of the spine, the axis and the atlas, cannot perform their function of delicately balancing the head. The next order was for the head to be directed forward and up—not *put* but directed.

The next order was to the back to lengthen and widen.

Alexander explained to us that this was the nearest he could get in words to the actuality he wished to bring about. These simple verbal formulations are designed to bring about the reconciliation of two opposing tendencies in each case, and to ensure the balance of forces in the antagonistic muscle pulls in the body. A harmony results, where everything is doing its own work of maintaining stability, and there is a stillness without fixity, or if you like, a lack of disturbance, in the working of the parts of the body in their relationship to each other.

Too much forward of the head and you lose the upward tendency —too much up and the head goes back—"leave it alone, in fact".

Too much effort to lengthen the back and it narrows—too much widening and you lose length and slump down.

The whole process is self-checking. I hope this makes clear why one cannot *do* the orders. Their first function is preventive. The wrong inner patterns are *the doing* which has to be stopped.

I'm afraid I have rather laboured this story—so familiar to many of the audience. The full account of it is in Alexander's book, *The Use of the Self*, but I warned you that I was going to re-examine our origins. It was necessary to do this if what follows is to make any sense, especially to our guests who may not know Alexander's teaching.

After he had worked out the technique by putting it into practice to restore his own normal co-ordination, he was very surprised to find that the misuses he had overcome in himself were present, in varying degrees, in everyone else.

It is a curious fact that until the scales fall from our eyes in this matter of misuse, we do not notice the misuse of others. It is as if the words about the beam in our eyes and the mote in other people's went into reverse.

Alexander then had to find a way of teaching others what he knew. This was a considerable task, involving not only explanation, but learning the special and subtle skill in the use of his hands needed for working on other people.

Later still he took on a further burden in the shape of students wanting to learn how to teach the work. This is a different task again, group work instead of work with one individual.

It is important to remember that we are all in the same situation as Alexander. He has found the way and the technique for following the way. We have the enormous advantage of the skilled help of a trained teacher. But the real importance and value of the technique is that we learn to work on ourselves.

Alexander used to say, "Everyone must do the *real* work for themselves. The teacher can show the way, but cannot get inside the pupil's brain and control his reactions for him. Each person must apply it for himself."

Learning this work is like learning anything else. We make use of the same faculties and need the same patience and perseverance as in any form of learning.

So far we have explored Alexander's work in its application to our faulty muscular habits and general misuse of the body, and seen how we may build up a stable good use which is under our control.

Let us now examine some applications of his principles to other spheres of our experience, and see if we can catch some part of the vision of its importance which inspired him throughout his life.

He understood, as perhaps no one else has done, that here was the possibility of a different quality of living, which could help resolve many of the difficulties of life which we bring on ourselves through lack of awareness and control. He was very modest about his part in the discoveries, and often used to say, "If I had not discovered the work some other poor chap would have had to go through all that, because the need for it is so great." This attitude is probably common among creative people. Once the poem is written, the music composed, the painting finished or the scientific discovery made, the creation assumes its own life, and its originator feels a certain detachment towards it.

The Alexander Technique will work wherever it is applied. It is not magic, but does its job at the point of application. How deeply it is applied depends on the aims and wishes of the person concerned. If the aim is to get rid of a pain in the back it will do so effectively by bringing into consciousness the "wrong doing" which is producing the pain. If the aim is greater awareness of habitual reactions in other departments of the self, it will work there too, and by the same process. We are all bound in the prison of habit. We have habits of thought—unexamined fixed opinions and prejudices which determine our behaviour without our realizing it.

We are also victims of habits of emotional reaction. These are very powerful driving forces.

A young pupil of my husband's, when she first realized the importance of these things, burst out, "Oh, I see, Dr Barlow, this is a life-sentence."

Alexander's favourite way of describing his work was "as a means of controlling human reaction". Under this basic umbrella can be included every form of blind, unconscious reaction, and here we come to the whole question of self-knowledge.

The muscular bad habits of misuse harm only oneself—unconscious habits of thought and emotion harm oneself *and* other people, because they determine our reactions to everyone else. It could be said that we use other people to practise our unconscious bad habits on.

The greatest misery and misunderstanding we experience is often in this field of personal relationships. Of course, these inner emotional states are mirrored in the way we use ourselves—states of rage, anxiety and fear—to take only the most obvious examples—are there for all the world to see by the unmistakable bodily attitudes. This is also true of more subtle inner conditions such as depression, worry and hopelessness.

In some ways the constant and deep reaction-patterns are more obvious to other people than to ourselves.

I sometimes think that there is a wry sense of humour lurking somewhere in the background of the Universe permitting this tragi-comic state of affairs, where certain characteristics of a person are known and clearly seen by everyone, except the person himself.

There is a thing known as "the state of the world". In whatever part of time a man's life-span is set down there must always be large, terrifying problems, known as the "state of the world".

In primitive times wild animals and marauding tribes were probably the main worries—apart from the weather. Later, perhaps, the plague, persecutions, lawlessness and lack of respect for human life. In this things haven't changed much—and always there is war.

An individual can do little about these large issues. On a smaller scale, but nearer home, there is the problem of other people. Most of the time they just don't behave as we think they should. Again there is little that we can do about it, although we waste an enormous amount of energy trying to make them alter.

Where then can we affect anything? We have been told many times in the course of history, by wise men, that the chaos in the world is only a reflection of the chaos within us—writ large.

Alexander taught that there is one main field of work for each of us —work on ourselves to gain more light on our unconscious habits— work to use more constantly the one place of freedom we have, the moment of the impact on us of a stimulus, so that we increase the number of moments when we *choose* our reaction, instead of being driven by habit to react as we have always done in the past. For this we must be *there*—present and aware, at the crucial moment, to inhibit before we react.

We have no freedom in dictating the state of the world, we have only limited control over the events that happen to us, but can develop control over the way we react to these events.

The freedom in our environment and in regard to other people's reactions is also limited, but we *can* have some control over the nearest bit of our environment—ourselves.

Alexander used to chide us for always trying to change and control the big things instead of changing the small things that were in our control. The inscription at Delphi "Know thyself" sums it up.

Down the ages we can see that all the real teachers of mankind have tried to make people understand this point, that change can only happen in the individual. We know that fundamental new ideas have always started with one person and spread slowly and gradually as more and more *individuals* receive and understand the new knowledge.

The vision Alexander had of the possibility of individual evolution in the development of consciousness and awareness was the mainspring of his life's work. It is this aspect of his teaching that places him in the direct tradition of the great teachers of humanity. It is this side of his teaching which could so easily get lost. It is a not unreasonable supposition that many whose reported teachings have come down to us, also gave to the people of their time practical techniques for carrying out the teaching. If so, most of this has been lost and forgotten, and we are left with reports and writings which today often have little meaning for us. It is interesting—apropos of all this—that a pupil of mine, a doctor, once remarked that Alexander had rediscovered the secret of Zen for our time.

Another aspect of traditional teaching worth mentioning is the necessity to live in the present. It is a recurrent theme in the great mystical writings. The Now is all that we have. We cannot inhibit next week, direct ourselves tomorrow, or even control our reactions five minutes hence. All this has to be done Now. The fact that we find it so difficult to BE in the present, and to deal with the requirements of the present moment in the most appropriate way is, I might suggest somewhat fancifully, also mirrored in the way we stand. How can we BE all present and correct, if our heads are driving back into the past, our bodies rushing forward into the future and only our feet all too firmly anchored in the Here and Now?

But you may say, Let's not be so gloomy about it, and, of course, you would be quite right. Nothing is achieved by gloom and heaviness. As one of our students pointed out, "If there is a force of gravity there must also be a force of levity."

Frequently, when he was training us, Alexander would come into the students' room, look around at all the earnest, serious faces preparing diligently for his class, and send us packing for a walk round the square saying, "That's not the way to work, let's have a bit of gaiety and lightness."

One of the most endearing things about him was his capacity for enjoyment and his refusal to be serious about things which did not really matter. He liked particularly jokes against himself and would tell them with great gusto. He knew the meaning of the words "enjoy yourself".

In 1946 my husband and I were on holiday in Brittany with Alexander and a South African QC with rather expensive tastes. We were nearing the end of our stay and were awaiting, rather anxiously, the arrival of some travellers cheques belonging to the South African. They did not come and, meanwhile, the rest of the party were supplying him with cash.

On the last day the cheques still hadn't arrived and we had 1,600 francs between us to foot a large hotel bill. After consultation we decided that the only thing to do was to send Alexander to the Casino in the hope that he would retrieve our fortunes. We all went with him and stood behind his chair while he, with the greatest composure in the world, proceeded very slowly and diligently to lose every sou that we had. As he remarked in another context, "You cannot change the course of Nature by primarily co-ordinating yourself."

All ended happily enough as Alexander had made friends with a young French couple who were staying in the hotel, and they agreed to stand surety for us until we could collect the money from the nearest large town.

But to return to his teaching. It is, like al important things, invisible and fragile, the heart and core of it I mean. There is a nice little piece by Rilke which I can't resist quoting, "This is the creature that has never been, they never knew it, yet, nonetheless, they loved the way it moved—its gentleness—its neck, its very gaze, calm and serene." I am reminded also of Bernard Shaw's remark, "Alexander calls upon the world to witness a change so small and so subtle that only he can see it."

Alexander's teaching comes into being—it is born anew, only when someone uses it. In this way it is like music, it is brought to life when someone plays it and makes the music manifest.

Alexander used to tell us that he wrote his books to ensure that a record of his work would exist if the teaching of it died out. His hope was, that in this event, someone might come across the books and reconstruct the practical side of it. Now, I know that these books come in for a lot of criticism. It has always been so. They are not easy to read and certainly they were not easy to write. But there they are—the man's own words—how he worked the problem out and what he thought his discoveries meant.

Francis Bacon said, "Some books are to be tasted, others to be swallowed, and some few to be chewed and digested."

I suggest that Alexander's books are obligatory reading for anyone who takes his teaching seriously.

He is accused of being incomprehensible. I would like to quote a passage from a recently translated book by Merlacu Ponty called *The Phenomenology of Perception.* "The excitation is seized upon and re-organised to make it resemble the perception which it is about to cause," end of quote.

I don't pretend to know what the author means, but I'm sure he is trying to express something important. It might even be worthwhile studying his book to find out. So with Alexander's books—they require study and hard application, given this they will yield up their gold.

Before the war I had a pupil who was home on leave from army service in India. He had a course of lessons and went back to his unit. Two or more years later he returned to London for a refresher course of lessons. I congratulated him on the change in himself which he had brought about. "Yes," he said, "I have been working hard. One thing has helped me more than anything else. I keep Alexander's books on my bedside table and read a chapter every night."

The following day I told Alexander this story while we were having a training class. He was silent for a long moment and then said thoughtfully, "Yes, and I would be a better man if I did the same."

These then are the two aspects of Alexander's teaching. First as a means of allowing the natural laws of the organism to work without interference—a means of giving back the birth-right of good use, which, as children, we all possessed. Alexander said, "When an investigation comes to be made it will be found that every single thing we do in the work is exactly what is done in Nature, where the conditions are right, the difference being that we are learning to do it consciously."

Ideally, the teacher has to be a craftsman in the use of his hands, a scientist in his adherence to principles which are subject to "operational verification" and an artist in conveying his knowledge to others.

The teacher's responsibility for the continued existence of the work is heavy, especially if he trains other teachers, to ensure that none of the essential elements of the teaching are lost.

In the second aspect—the application of the work to deeper spheres of our experience, the division into teacher and pupil vanishes.

There is no end to work on oneself—here we are all in the same boat.

When Alexander was nearly 80 years old he said to me, "I never stop working on myself—I dare not." He knew that the only limits to this kind of development are those which we impose on ourselves.

He continued to teach to within five days of the end, at the age of 86 and then, having refused all drugs which might deprive him of it, he achieved the rare distinction of being present at his own death.

Tonight we have remembered him—but the memorial that would please *him* best is that we should do his work.

TWO

A Diary of Lessons with Alexander
by Louise Morgan

AN OLD AMERICAN friend of mine, Miss G. R., of New York, turned up in London after several years' absence. She was so much altered in appearance that it gave me a shock. Never have I seen such a deterioration in any human being. Her figure as I recalled it was slender and upright, her complexion clear and bright, and she was always full of energy, with quick darting movements. But now her head was sunk between her shoulders, her skin had the look of old parchment, she had grown stout and round-shouldered, one leg dragged, and she could stand only with the help of a stick. She had not walked for months. Only a spark of her old spirit was left. She made a gallant attempt to be gay, but the moment she ceased struggling her face became almost a death mask.

The story she told me was the tragic one of failure to recover properly from a serious disease, and gradual lapse into invalidism. She had seen specialist after specialist, faithfully following all that was prescribed for her, only to grow slowly but steadily worse. Fortunately for her, she had a fairly substantial income, so she was able to travel to London for what she called "final consultations". I thought of suggesting that she first consult Alexander, and I eventually succeeded in persuading her to see him. I felt sure he could help her, and must have conveyed my feeling of certainty to her. She did see him, and was so impressed by his personality that she decided to make a final effort to save herself, and put herself entirely in his hands.

A few days later I accompanied her to her lesson and from that day until she was obliged to return home to New York seven weeks later, I kept in close touch with her. We talked over her lessons, and discussed Alexander's philosophy. She began to read his books, and became so interested that she kept a diary of her lessons. She has given me permission to quote certain parts of it. It tells the story so well that I shall allow it to speak for itself. It is the first diary on the subject of the Alexander Technique to be published. I think it provides an excellent introduction to the technique as well as a heartening and inspiring human record.

A Diary of Lessons

Third lesson: I notice that Alexander keeps giving my knees a gentle tap to remind me not to stiffen them unduly and not to hold them rigid. He also taps my ribs to remind me to keep them moving. Joints must be free, he says, and ribs must constantly expand and contract for good breathing. I feel he is trying to show me how to keep my head up out of my shoulders, to keep it forward and up. He is also trying to lengthen my back and my spine upward, and to raise up all parts of me that have been pressed down. I feel he is remodelling my back. I don't seem to be able to do much myself, but I hope to co-operate with him soon. Something has begun to happen to me at last. It is a bit tiring, but something is happening, and that's the great thing.

Fourth lesson: How hard A. works. His hands seem to fly about trying to help me keep my head up out of my shoulders and keep it forward and up. He tells me not to do anything about it, but just to think it, but I don't get the point. There must be a point, and I must learn what it is. He seems to know exactly what to do, and never hesitates a moment. I am certain he knows what to do, unlike all the others who have tried out such awful things on me. I am certain he will never hurt me, so I have no fear of him. He makes me feel calm and happy and interested. He is trying to lengthen my back and my spine, the poor crooked things. That great hand of his seems to cover my whole back, guiding the muscles to lift me. "And the crooked thing shall be made straight." I want to co-operate, but still feel a bit helpless. I can hardly move.

Seventh lesson: I am still struggling to grasp Alexander's new ideas. He is right. You have to keep a very open mind if you are his pupil. It seems that I am letting my head go back even when I feel I am keeping it forward. He says it's most important for me to keep my head from going back, because it interferes with the "primary control"—whatever that is. I must read his book to find out. It appears to be something in the region of the neck and head, where they join together, which controls the working of the whole muscular system. I have always been for central control—that is, putting one person at the head of a department and making them responsible for it and not interfering with them. Maybe it's something like that. Alexander does say the primary control makes for wonderful efficiency and harmony. We shall see. Or at least, I hope I shall see! How I do go on about all this. But I just can't help being interested.

It's one of the most fascinating things I've ever struck. Where was I? Oh yes, putting my head back when I feel I am keeping it forward and up. Alexander says this is because the habit of putting it back is so strong that it feels right for me to put it back, and wrong to keep it forward. He also mentioned "faulty sensory perception", but I don't get this yet.

I am now remembering pretty well to keep my ribs moving and my knees free. He is still working away on my head, neck and shoulders, with an occasional heave-up of my back that makes me feel as if I'd grown a yard. I feel so confident and full of power when he puts my head right and keeps it there, as if I could walk right round the block. But then I let my head go back, and the power leaves me flat. I am not depressed, but I feel I am a long way out on a very weak limb.

Ninth lesson: Beginning to see light on feeling. It appears that what feels right may be very wrong. All the things which feel right for me to do are wrong. So I must not do the wrong thing—that is, the thing that to me feels right. Sounds fantastic, but actually I'm beginning to see it's not in the least fantastic. I put my head back, naturally because I have always done it, and so it feels right. But putting my head back is wrong because I can do nothing right when it is back. It interferes with that "primary control"! This all boils down to the fact that I must STOP doing the thing that FEELS right to me.

Today I realize how short I had grown without knowing it. My back curved in at the middle, and shortened my spine. It happened so gradually that I did not realize it. When I take good breaths by moving my ribs a lot, I notice that this makes me feel taller. (I really must be careful about this word "feel"! Maybe I'm not so tall as I feel!) If I might presume to suggest it, some of the trouble is that we often say "think" when we mean "feel", and say "feel" when we mean "think". My brain is very active these days, as if it was waking up from a nice refreshing nap. This is one of the best signs of the good Alexander is doing me. Alexander said today that when one breathes the right way, one lengthens the spine and widens and strengthens the back. He is pleased with the way I keep my ribs moving and my knees free. My poor old knees! I don't feel a spark of life in them sometimes. Thank goodness I can do something, even if I can't understand these new ideas as well as I should like.

Eleventh lesson: Alexander still saying "Don't do anything you feel is right". Drat feelings! They are low-down, sneaky things that creep up on you and "cosh" you. All the same he seemed pleased with me today. Several times I managed to stop before doing anything, say "No" to my feeling, and think the way to do right. And I DID right. It's really indescribable when you can stop doing a wrong thing and do a right thing instead, just by thinking. I stopped getting up wrong and got up right, and I KNEW I could do it. Alexander is showing me how to change a bad habit into a good one. You change it by stopping the old feeling and learning a new one. I hope I can hang on to this idea, and never forget it. I believe I'm writing all this down to remind me of these new things. I kept my head forward and up pretty nearly all the time today. Towards the end of the lesson Alexander put his fingertips, only two of them, at the base of my head, and I stood up like a breeze. Then he asked me to stand up again, and again, and each time I got up better than I had ever done in my life. Better than I had done when I was well, before that awful illness. I always used to haul myself more or less ungracefully out of a chair, and used to wonder how ballet dancers managed to rise up so beautifully. It gave me a thrill to realize that I was doing something better than when I was perfectly well. But the best of it was yet to come. Alexander said "I don't know whether you know, but you did the last two all by yourself. I didn't help you in any way. I kept my finger-tips an inch away from your neck." Marvel of marvels. I got out of a chair all by myself for the first time in years—"did it twice". This was a red letter day.

Twelfth lesson: Not so good. I guess I got too excited yesterday over my success, and was careless. I seem to have slipped back into the old habit of use of myself again. I just couldn't do a thing right. I mean, wrong! Which reminds me that I've enjoyed myself more, and laughed more, since I came to Alexander, than in years. He comforted me by saying that I can't expect to wipe out years of misuse in twelve lessons. I must hold this thought over me. It's wonderful, a miracle, what has happened to me in twelve lessons. It's happened in my brain as well as my body.

I have been feeling new aches and pains. I've been such a mass of discomfort and misery for so long that I don't much notice them. But there is no doubt that they are NEW ones. My muscles are changing over. Of course they shout about it. Bound to. My "dead" leg seems stiffer than ever, and more lifeless. He says very little these days, though we usually have a crack or two. He just works and works on my head, neck and back. I even let my knees go stiff today and forgot to move my ribs. I also put my arms out when I started to get up, an

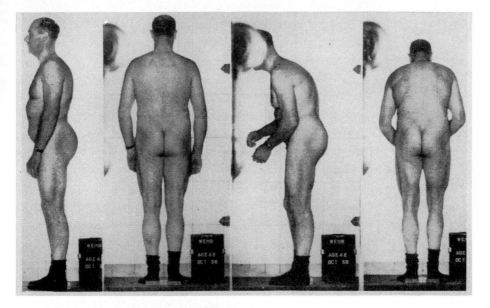

1. (*above*) Pastry Cook from side and back, and stooping forward over work

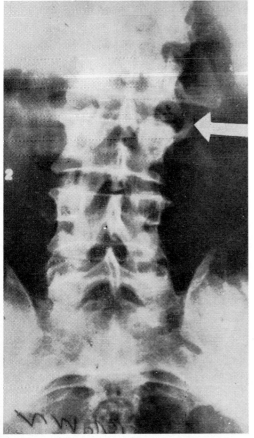

2. (*left*) Arrow indicating osteophyte

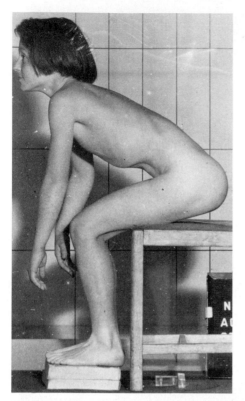

3. (*left*) Head pulled back, body thrown forward, pelvis thrown back

4. (a) (*below, left*) Repeated extension movement in hysteric. Such muscular over-contraction interferes with the body-schema by cutting out muscle-spindle afferent impulses

4. (b) (*below, right*) Similar extension movement mistakenly employed by physio-therapists in postural re-education

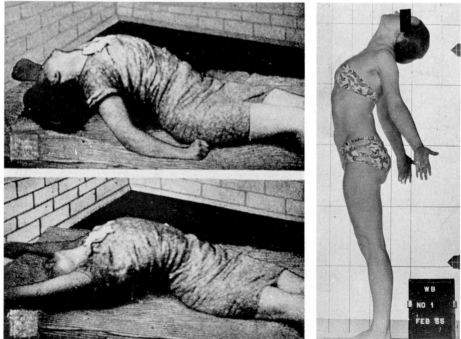

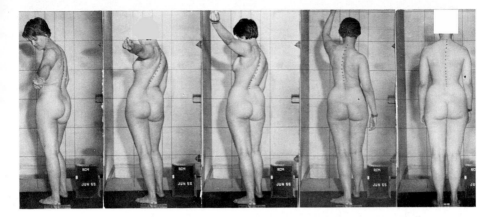

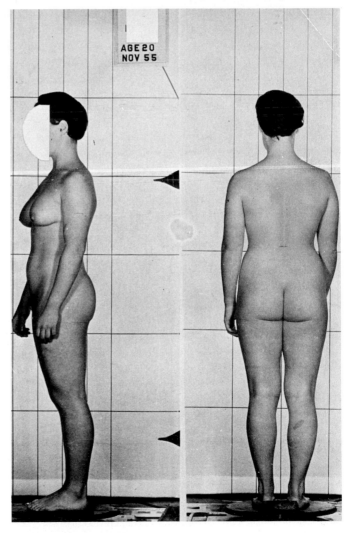

AGE 20
NOV 55

5. (*above*) Left-handed javelin-thrower, showing development of lateral curvature during movement

6. (*right*) Rotation of right shoulder and breast

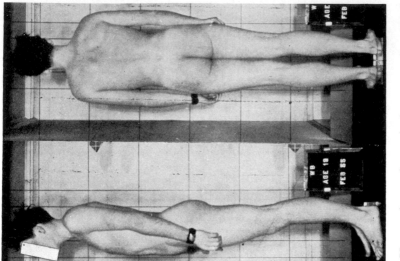

7. Identical twins with identical mis-use. Notice dropped right shoulder and tension right side of neck

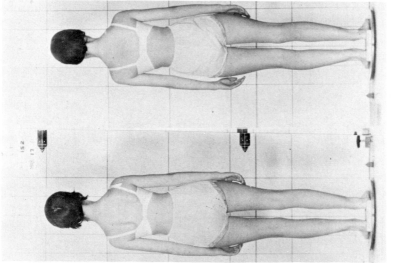

8. Unconscious pain-producing contraction of left shoulder

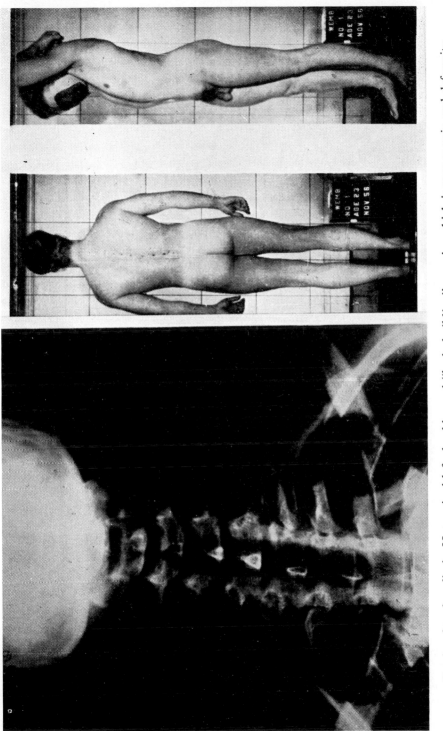

9. Cervico-dorsal scoliosis. Note raised left shoulder and "body-building" exercise which increases pain and deformity

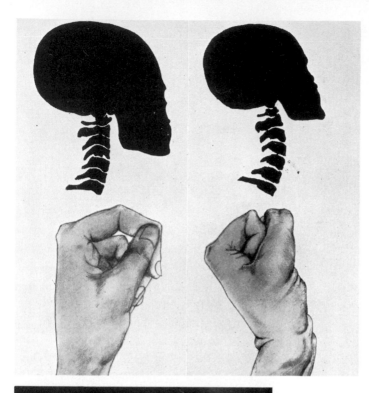

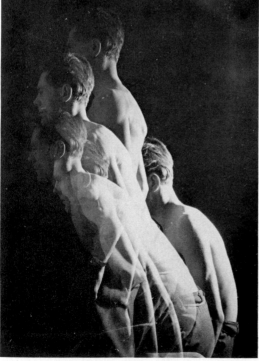

10. (*above*) Movement at wrist indicating head retraction. Cervical lordosis corrected by movement similar to wrist movement

11. (*left*) Head retraction when standing up

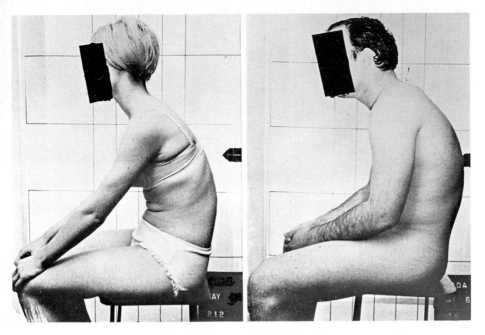

12. Typical slumped sitting positions

13. Three sitting positions: (a. *left*) slumping; (b. *centre*) sitting too straight; and (c. *right*) balanced

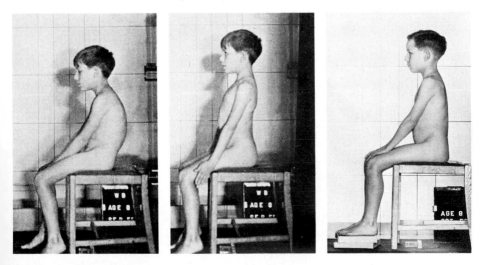

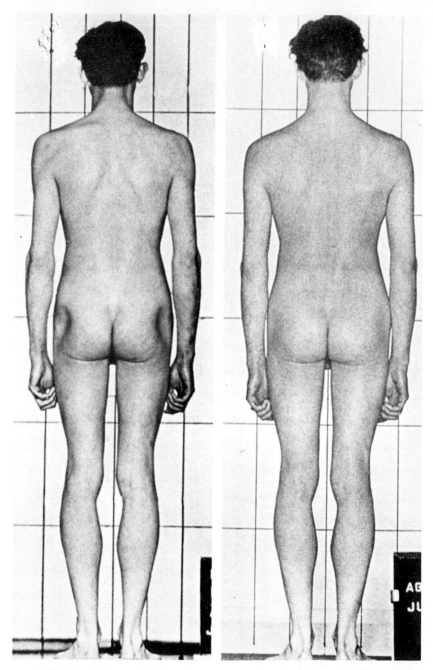

14. Posture before (*left*) and after (*right*) Alexander training. The photograph shows muscle contractions at the back of the neck; raised shoulders and tightened buttocks. After training, these tensions had disappeared and the patient was overall taller

awful thing to do which I haven't done for some time. But am I depressed? No fear!

Sixteenth lesson: The new aches and pains still go on. Now my leg is badder than ever. But Alexander has no pity on me. He says, "Splendid!" when I tell him I ache all over. He even tells me he is glad to hear that I'm stiffer and achier and sorer! Seriously, I see that it means good things are happening to me. The old muscle pattern is changing. No, I am changing my muscle pattern! Just like that. Grand, isn't it! If it only means that I can throw away that stick one day. I don't mind what I go through! It may be that I expect too much because I get so much. To compensate me for a rather poor lesson today the hotel porter says he thinks I'm looking much better and brighter, and almost like my old self. Dear old chap he knew me when I was well. My mirror tells me that my skin has improved a lot. I am sleeping lots better too. I am really much better inside myself. So here goes for a good lesson tomorrow. But bother that stiffness and soreness!

Eighteenth lesson: Another new idea. Would you believe it! I am giving orders to my brain. I am saying to it, "Tell my muscles not to do this," and "Tell my muscles to do that." Changing habit by changing message-paths in the brain. I say "Stop" to myself, or to my brain, and stop certain old processes. Then I say to myself, "Head forward and up, neck relaxed, spine lengthening, back widening." I don't DO anything, but just think it. Next thing I know I am on my feet without the least effort. This, says Alexander, comes of thinking not of DOING but of the MEANS-WHEREBY one can achieve what one wants. This "means-whereby" seems to be very important. I don't get it yet, but I guess I will in time. Anyway, it works!! So, instead of concentrating on getting up gracefully without a jerk or a jump, I think about the means-whereby I can do it. And then I do it. All Alexander's ideas seem to work together in some mysterious way. They make their own kind of sense. I shall see the whole pattern one day. He has thoroughly i-dotted and t-crossed everything. I guess this will do for one lesson.

Nineteenth lesson: All through my lessons Alexander has never stopped tapping me lightly with his fingertips to remind me of things I should keep doing. It works out very well, because even in the hotel at night I feel that light tap, and change to the new use of myself. He taps my ribs to remind me about the new use of myself in breathing,

B

my knees to remind me not to keep them stiff, and my neck near the head to remind me to keep my head forward and up.

I am trying to free all my joints, which seem as if they were set in concrete. They are stiff as boards; but in general it seems to me that the old kind of stiffness is going. Touch wood. (My knees will do!) I now always remember to stop getting up wrong, and to think of the means-whereby I can get up right. But I don't always get up successfully because I don't always keep my head forward and up. Alexander is right in all he says. I have found that it is quite impossible for me to get up out of a chair without a jump if I have put my head back. I just know that if I have not come up in one smooth movement, I've got my head back. This is something I know, and will never forget. I've learned it inside myself, by the changes that are going on inside myself. I am beginning to see how the "means-whereby" tied up with keeping my head forward and up.

Twentieth lesson: Whew! what a lesson! My cheeks were quite rosy when I got back, and I hardly knew myself. The porter said, "It won't be long now before you're walking without my help." Usually it takes both him and his second in command to get me from my taxi to my room. Alexander began by showing me how amazingly flexible his joints are. Each separate part of his fingers seems to be coming out of its joint, and his hand seems to be coming out of the wrist joint, and his forearm out of the elbow joint. Such suppleness, like elastic! How I envy him his supple joints. They make his hands soft as a breeze yet strong as steel. I told him he would have made a wonderful acrobatic dancer, and it made him roar. I may say that by now, I am pretty good at getting up from the chair without a jump. But never until today have I succeeded in sitting down without a powerful bump. His theme song used to be "Don't jump". Lately it's been "Don't bump". I get about a third of the way down all right, and then I become anxious and put my head back. And so I flop down with a bump. But today praise heaven, I sat down as if on air. I wasn't able to repeat it, but just that once it was glorious. I felt like singing a hymn of thanksgiving. Never, never shall I forget that moment. I have done it once, so I shall be able to do it again. This getting up and sitting down like a feather has shown me what an awful state I have slipped into. That illness got me down pretty low, and I've been sinking lower and lower ever since without realizing it. Doctors don't seem to realize what a long illness can do to you, and how much help you need to get back your health! No trouble is too much to be able to stand up and sit down in this wonderful way, as if I owned the earth, and the world was my oyster, and so on. Just to think that I can do this in only twenty lessons of only half an hour each, when the doctors have worked on me for years. This lesson is the best I've had. Alexander said when I got out of the chair (that dear old Queen Anne chair!), "That, my dear lady, was perfection personified." I beamed like a Cheshire cat. What a lesson! I simply can't wait for the next.

Twenty-sixth lesson: Last night, while loosening my knee joints, I felt life in my "dead" leg for the first time. I could hardly believe it at first, but it was there all right. I gave the great news to Alexander first thing, but all he said was "Good", quite calmly, as if he were taking it for granted. I suppose really he knows what is going on inside me better than I do myself. But if his leg had been like a piece of cast iron, and suddenly began to move, I bet he would have made a song and dance about it. Today I was expecting wonders, but I got up right about ten times and got up wrong ten times. Maybe this is what you call progress (well, I can still laugh), I go over my lessons every day in the hotel, trying to do what he expects of me. By the way, it no longer exhausts me to write. My hand and my brain both feel pretty fresh when I finish my diary, instead of being worn out. Today we talked again about the wrong habit of giving the right feeling and about saying "Stop" or "No" to it each time you want to do something. Experience has proved to me that this is absolutely true. It does work every time. Lord knows how he discovered it. All I have to do is put this truth into action. My leg felt alive during this lesson, but I was careful not to boast about it. I'm not out of the woods yet, so I must not crow too much. I'll keep my thrills about my "Dead" leg to myself.

Forgot to note that I've had lessons while lying on a table. I am told to "think the knees going up to the ceiling", and I do so. It seems to loosen the joints without any effort on my part except the thinking. I can't raise the "dead" leg yet without help, but once it's up I can hold it there. When I lie on the table I have a book under my head like a Chinese lady of long ago. It helps me keep my head from going back. Alexander still goes on tapping my ribs, knees and neck to remind me. This helps a lot.

Thirtieth lesson: I have been sleeping much better and my waist-line is beginning to appear again. Still rather full of stiffness, but it is definitely less. Alexander says today, "I can see your improvement in the better colour of your skin." That is good to hear, and confirms what the porter said. I'm really lucky to have found Alexander. Why doesn't everybody know about him? This is the kind of thing we all need, I'm certain, even the healthy ones among us. It seems crazy that he should not be as famous as so many men are who don't do half what he does for the good of humanity. It's the same story today that we've repeated so often. Alexander working on my head, neck, shoulders and back, and me attending to my means-whereby I still keep getting up and sitting down. I thought of the people who have sat in that Queen Anne chair. The great G.B.S. sat in it for 40 lessons and did just the same things I am trying to do. It is quite an inspiring reflection. Nice to think that I can do some of the things Shaw did, even though I couldn't write *Man and Superman*.

Thirty-second lesson: I AM Taller. I have measured myself. I noticed that when I looked out the hotel window before putting my head forward and up, I saw less of the scene from the bottom than when I looked out with my head forward and up. Then I tried looking out before giving myself orders, and while looking out I gave myself the orders, and was delighted to find the scene rising before my very eyes, The picture seemed to come up inches above the window-sill and I saw yards more of the buildings across the street. It was quite a dramatic discovery, but I did not tell Alexander I worked it out for myself that the curves in my back are straightening out, therefore giving me more height. I also know that my old porter seems less tall to me than when I arrived here. So I actually am taller. At the end of today's lesson I walked from the chair to the sofa without my stick. I took it in small steps. But I did walk by myself. Now I know that I shall walk again. No one will know what this means to me except someone who has gone through the same experience. It is impossible to describe what walking on one's feet can mean to a person who has not walked for years. It is a miracle to me. I'm getting used to miracles. I just hold my breath, cross my fingers, praise God and wait for the next one to happen.

At that point the diary breaks off. Miss G. R. had an urgent call back to New York owing to a family emergency. She had two or three more lessons, but there was no time to write about them. In these, Alexander gave her instructions about how she was to carry on until she could return. I had several talks with her as she did her packing and made arrangements for her return in six months' time. It was good to see her walking round the room—a bit carefully, of course. But all the same, walking. She seemed again like her old self. Gone was the strained, deathly look, the humped-over back, the dragging leg. No longer did she suggest an object of pity.

In our last talk, she suddenly said, "I suppose you realize that Alexander has saved my life. I was returning home less than three months ago to prepare myself for death. Oh, nothing dramatic, but just to put my affairs in order. I'm going home a new person, ready to start a new life. What a teacher he is! He should be teaching the whole world."

THREE

In the Supreme Court of South Africa
(Witwatersrand Local Division)

Before the Honourable Mr Justice Clayden

Appearances:
Mr J. H. Hanson, KC, with Mr A. Fischer, for the Plaintiff, Frederick Matthias Alexander.
Mr O. Pirow, KC, with Mr M. van Hulsteyn for the Defendants.

Opening Address

MR HANSON: "May it please your lordship. This is an action in which the plaintiff, Mr Frederick Matthias Alexander, of London, the founder of a technique which is known under his name, sues the defendants for £5,000 damages for defamation.

"I feel at this stage it would be proper to tell your lordship a little of the plaintiff, such as we will be able to prove in evidence, and something of his technique, something of his teachings, something of his books, so that your lordship, in the course of hearing the evidence, will be able to get a proper perspective of what the witness will talk about."

MR PIROW: "Permit me my lord. I take it my learned friend is outlining the evidence which either has been taken on commission in London or will be taken in this court, because beyond that there is nothing, I submit, which he can convey to your lordship."

HIS LORDSHIP: "That is presumably what he is doing."

MR PIROW: "I just want to make sure of that."

MR HANSON: "The books, of course, will be evidence before the court and I propose to address your lordship on some of the things that appeared in the books, so that your lordship can understand what the witnesses will talk about.

"The plaintiff, at the close of the last century, was an elocutionist carrying on his profession in Australia when he became afflicted with some throat trouble which involved him in the loss of his voice when any strain was thrown on it. He made a painstaking investigation into the cause of his trouble, because medical aid had failed. This investigation led him to the conclusion that the cause of his trouble lay in his own use of his organs connected with speaking and that the strain—just putting it briefly—on his larynx was caused by the misuse of his own head and neck. As a result of these investigations he further concluded that this misuse discovered in himself was prevalent among the peoples of his generation, and, eventually, in the course of his investigations, he evolved a theory and a technique which eventually established him as a teacher of his system, to re-educate persons in the use of themselves.

"Early in the century, in any event, some years prior to 1910, in circumstances which I will, unfortunately, be precluded from proving to this court, Mr Alexander had removed himself from Australia and had established himself in London, where he carried on his teaching, and since then he has done so for 40 years, save for a short interruption during the last war when his school for training young children had been bombed and he removed himself and his pupils to America until it was safe for him to return to England.

"Now, my lord, Mr Alexander is not simply a teacher of a technique. His researches have led him to ponder on the destiny of man in evolution, and Mr Alexander has elaborated a philosophy which has influenced, as I will hope to prove to your lordship, some at least of the thought of his day. In his career he published four books and I think I could at this stage hand your lordship these books in the order in which they appeared."

MR PIROW: "My learned friend should give your lordship all the editions; there are various editions, and we allege there are discrepancies in the various editions. If he is handing in books it may be that he can hand in copies of the various editions as well."

HIS LORDSHIP: "If you wish to do that."

MR HANSON: "No, my lord. I do not wish to do that. I do not happen to have sufficient copies of all the editions and no doubt my learned friend, at any proper time in this case, if he wants to, can do so. These are the books that were used when evidence was taken on commission. They used the 1946 editions."

HIS LORDSHIP: "Are these the 1946 editions?"

MR HANSON: "Yes, my lord. These books will be referred to by their titles and not by exhibit numbers. Your lordship will see that the first book that was written was named *Man's Supreme Inheritance*. That book first appeared in 1910. There have been a considerable number of editions since then, in 1918, 1937, 1939, 1941, and your lordship has the 1946 edition. The reason why I am giving your lordship the 1946 edition is that, when the evidence was taken in

London, particularly in relation to the witnesses called by the defendants, their references were made to the 1946 edition. It will prove much easier for your lordship to follow, at least in the evidence called on behalf of the defendants. The second book, *Constructive Conscious Control*, first appeared in 1923; the book called *The Use of the Self* first appeared in 1932; and *The Universal Constant in Living* first appeared in 1942. There were subsequent editions to these books. I do not think your lordship need worry about noting those dates."

HIS LORDSHIP: "No. But, I think, Mr Hanson, other copies of these books are going to be put in. It may be convenient at a later stage, if they were marked A, B, C, and D, so that if there is reference to any other edition, they may be identified."

MR HANSON: "It can only be referred to as the 1918 edition, and so on. Now, my lord, I would say at once that Mr Alexander has no pretensions to literary skill. The books are not advanced by him or by us in this case as models of composition or literary structure. But these four books do contain all the thoughts and theories which were provoked by Mr Alexander's observations and which formed, I might say, his philosophy. His technique, the technique of his teaching, which is a method of education, is based on that philosophy. And it is based, if I can put it shortly, on the evolution of man from an unconscious, unreasoning creature to a completely conscious individual.

"Now, his first book, *Man's Supreme Inheritance*, expounds his philosophy, and it is based on the conception of man as a psychophysical unit, that is, of mind on the physical side, as a unit. Briefly, his theme is as follows: That in the process of evolution man, as distinct from other animals, has developed a power of reasoning and has a quality of consciousness which distinguishes him from any of the lower animals. But man's destiny in the process of evolution was that his consciousness or his reason must play an ever increasing rôle in man's behaviour, both in his social relationships and in the manner in which man uses himself. His philosophy is this, that by virtue of man's reasoning or his consciousness, man has been able radically to change the environment in which he lives. To illustrate, my lord, the savage lived in primordial forests, on plains, and he supplied his needs directly from hunting and from contact with that environment. But through the ages, and with increasing rapidity in the last 100 years, man has developed from that primitive stage, and he has, by virtue of his reasoning, completely changed his environment. Today man does not live from hunting. The instincts that were sufficient for man when he hunted are, in modern times, quite insufficient. Man earns his living today sitting behind a desk in an office or working a machine or by thinking. His leisure is different from what it was. His locomotion is different from what it was. He has not to depend on the instincts with which he was originally endowed and which from time to time he improved by virtue of his environment. So that his theme is this, that the needs of man today are no longer capable of being satisfied by any instinctive process. Mr Alexander believes, and he observes in his books, that this change of environment has occurred so rapidly that it has completely outstripped man's ability to live naturally in his changed environment. Whereas once his instinct was a sufficient guide—at a time, of course, when man was more reliant on the physical side and less on the mental side—today that environment is not adequate.

"Now, Mr Alexander observes that in the process of evolution man's reasoning, both in relation to his environment and in relation to himself, has developed. The one has not been so rapid. The pace of his reasoning in relation to the use of himself has been slower than the rate in which he has applied his reasoning to his changing environment. And that originally, many thousands, tens of thousands of years ago, it was not difficult for a man to adapt his habits to the use of himself to the very gradual changes in his environment. And for a great deal of the period of man's evolution he was an adequately adjusted creature, using himself efficiently. But Alexander's theme is this, man's present environment, in all walks of life, both in his social relations, and in the use of himself, requires that man should be fully conscious of the way in which he uses himself, that is conscious as to how he uses himself as a thinking, acting entity. But man has not learnt the abilities to do so. Mr Alexander's observation is that though man has this capacity to apply his reasoning today he has not, at the present stage of evolution, the ability to do so; though he has the capacity, man today still relies upon what he calls his instinctive or habitual uses, which are quite inadequate.

"In the present age the human being, from early childhood to fully-developed adolescence, is not taught (we know it is so from our own lives) to be aware of himself and his manner of use. From childhood he acts in this sense unconsciously; he uses himself fortuitously or by unconscious imitation; he acquires certain habits and the manner in which the individual uses himself becomes habitual, and as Mr Alexander observes, in our times almost universally incorrectly. For instance, the child in its tender years when performing some function that it does daily, acquires a stoop over its work, or acquires a habit of hunching his shoulders every time he performs some act. That use becomes habitual to the child, and it grows into a man who will always walk about perhaps with one shoulder higher than the other, as I am endeavouring to imitate, or with a stoop in its posture. Mr Alexander has observed that that use, which has become habitual, feels to the individual natural and correct. The man who walks around with an unsightly stoop does not feel in himself that he is acting unnaturally or incorrectly; that has become to him the natural way he uses himself, a posture which, to him, feels correct and natural. Should you take that individual and put him in a different posture physically, by straightening him by the force of your hands, the new position would feel, says Mr Alexander (and there is a lot of evidence on this), strained, unnatural and incorrect.

"And he makes another very essential observation in his technique. You can take a child and stand it up straight, put its shoulders in the correct position or what appears to be in the correct position, not necessarily in the correct position, and the child will be able to maintain that position only momentarily while it is stationary, but the moment the child proceeds to some activity—or the adult for that matter—, goes to pick up something or proceeds to sit down, the old bad manner of use will assert itself. From standing straight the child, the moment it goes to pick up a toy, will revert to the stoop or to the one shoulder higher than the other as being the natural posture which it adopts in activity. And it is this quality in man which makes a crooked head feel straight. The individual who habitually carries his head on the one side, whose head is put straight, will feel that his head is on the other side and not straight. To the outside world, looking at the man, it will appear that his head is straight, to himself, his sensations will be that his head is leaning over to the side to which he is not accustomed.

"And that, my lord, is what Mr Alexander calls in his work 'the false sensory appreciation' of the man and it is a factor that he has had to cope with in evolving his technique and one which proved to Mr Alexander the great difficulty in teaching a man the correct use of himself and which led to the development of his technique. There is a very forceful illustration of this, which I think falls properly in my opening, so as to give your lordship a picture. In the book, *Conscious Control of the Individual*, at pages 90 and 91, where he describes a distorted child who was brought to him. He says this:

A little girl who had been unable to walk properly for some years was brought to the writer for a diagnosis of the defects and the use of the psycho-physical mechanisms, which were responsible for a more or less crippled state. When this had been done a request was made that a demonstration should be given to those present of the manipulative side of the work, the child, of course was to be the subject to be manipulated, so that certain adjustments and co-ordinations might be temporarily secured, thus, showing, in keeping with the diagnosis, the possibility of the education on a general basis in a case of this type. The demonstration was successful from this point of view. For the time being the child's body was comparatively straightened out, that is, without the extreme twists and distortions which had been so noticeable when she came into the room. When this was done the little girl looked across her shoulder and said in an indescribable tone: 'Mummy, he has pulled me out of shape.' It was for this reason that the child felt she was no longer in shape.

It was this particular feature, observed Mr Alexander, which proved to him the great difficulty in teaching a correctness to individuals which led to the development of his technique.

"This case will abound with evidence of this sort, that it is useless to order a person to *do* the correct thing; it is no good saying to a man who has developed a marked misuse of his body, 'Stand up straight,' because the feeling of the old incorrect manner will be a feeling that it was right and natural, and the man trying to do what is right, in the way Mr Alexander puts it, will not do what he feels to be wrong. A man who feels that he is standing wrongly, if he has a certain posture of the shoulders, who is trying to do the right thing, will not, when he sits down or when he walks, or when he proceeds to some activity, do it in what is the right way if he feels that way to be the wrong way.

"And that, my lord, is the first step in the teaching of this technique; the first step is to make the individual with the wrong use aware of what is wrong and to make him aware of what is right, that is, by conscious awareness. It can be done by demonstration; if his use is wrong; to show him, to appeal to his reason, as to what is the right way in which he should do it. Then, Mr Alexander's observation is, that, to teach the pupil to acquire an habitual use of what is right, the first quality that the pupil must be taught is an ability to prevent, to inhibit himself from doing what is wrong; he must inhibit his natural reaction and he must prevent himself from responding to a stimulus to act at all, because it is action which brings into operation his habitual misuses. If I might explain that.

A man learning the technique is ordered to sit. If he obeys the order he will immediately use himself in his old wrong way, because he cannot help himself; he feels right; he feels natural. The thing he must do to the order to sit is to inhibit, prevent himself, when obeying that order, from using himself the wrong way; the pupil must then be given the experience of correct use by the means that Mr Alexander will give him. But he must not respond to the order to sit if his fault has been to bring his head back or hunch his shoulders; he would immediately fall into that posture if he were not all the time consciously inhibiting his response to the stimulus.

"That, my lord, is the second step of Mr Alexander's technique about the necessity for the pupil to inhibit. It is a prime conception in his teaching. At the same time, while the pupil is inhibiting in the teaching of the technique, the experiences of the correct use must be given by the teacher. The pupil himself must do nothing but inhibit, and the teacher will, by this teacher's hand, move the pupil in the correct way, so that the pupil will acquire, not at once but in time, the new sense, the new feeling of the correct use. And briefly, my lord, without going into all the obstacles that present themselves in teaching, Mr Alexander says that, although this use will at first feel wrong and unnatural, the person feeling wrong and out of shape, in some cases feeling discomfort and may even feel pain, after sufficient repetition at the hands of a teacher, the correct use will come to him to feel right and natural and will become consciously the habitual use of the pupil, replacing his old, unconscious habitual incorrect use.

"Now, my lord, I would like to say to your lordship that these ideas and methods of Mr Alexander have not passed unnoticed in the scientific field. Evidence will be given to your lordship that, many years after Mr Alexander wrote his first book, Sir Charles Sherrington, acknowledged—there is no dispute about this—acknowledged on all hands to be the greatest living physiologist of our time and today a man of over 90 years of age, makes reference to these concepts and teachings of Alexander in his latest work, *The Endeavour of Jean Fernel*, a work which appeared subsequent to the libel in this case, but, fortunately, before the hearing of the case, otherwise Mr Alexander might have found himself even in greater difficulties in getting some scientific support for the ideas that he had been working on for 50 years. Sir Charles Sherrington has this passage,—and I believe that it is not inappropriate to read it at this stage, because it will put much of what is said in a proper setting. Perhaps I should direct your lordship's attention to the fact that Sir Charles

Sherrington uses language very similar to Mr Alexander's and shows
that in fact he has taken a deal of it from Mr Alexander's language.
Speaking of human acts, Sir Charles Sherrington says this:

> Our attention is directed to the 'aim' of the act, not to the 'how' of
> it; the 'how' often enough takes care of itself. Conscious effort
> would seem unable to put us in touch actually with the propriocep-
> tive reflex itself. So illusive is this last that for long our muscles
> were unrecognized as affording any sensual basis of our motor acts.
> When we bend a finger we can, without looking at the finger and
> without the finger touching anything, tell within a little how
> much or how little we bend it; no hint, however, is vouchsafed
> to us that muscles doing the act lie up the forearm, or of the
> tensions or lengths they assume in doing it. When we turn our
> gaze we are not aware of the muscles of our eyeballs, nor can
> any mental effort or intensity of purpose make us so. Nonetheless,
> the unconscious reflexes at work in them are indispensable
> to the due performance of our act. In evolutionary history,
> behaviour such as that part of our own which Descartes relegated
> to 'reason' and 'free will', seems of later development than is
> the robot behaviour, operated reflexly. . . . Descended from a
> long stock of less mentalized creatures as we are, and living less
> reflexly than they did, our more mentalized status has arrived at
> putting the reflex mechanism as a going concern, within the
> control, to a certain extent, of the reactions of the brain. The
> mastery of the brain over the reflex machinery does not take the
> form of intermeddling with reflex details; rather it dictates to a
> reflex mechanism 'you may act' or 'you may not act'. The
> detailed execution of the motor act is still in immediate charge of
> the reflex. Our individual history exemplifies this.

"I hope, my lord, that when the case is developed much further
than it is now your lordship will appreciate that that is Mr Alexander's
teaching, namely, that consciously you can direct the manner of your
use; you can direct whether the reflex pattern should work or should
not work; you can adjust yourself so that the reflex action will work
properly, put in scientific terms. Then, of course, what happens with
reflex actions you cannot control. You cannot control whether you
shall digest or not digest, or whether your liver will function or not
function. But if you use yourself properly—if you do not interfere
with the reflex patterns as Mr Alexander teaches—the automatic
functions will function better.

"Sir Charles Sherrington goes on to say:

It is largely the reflex element in the willed movement or posture which, by reason of its unconscious character, defeats our attempts to know the 'how' of the doing of even a willed act. Breathing, standing, walking, sitting, although innate, along with our growth, are apt, as movements, to suffer from defects in our ways of doing them. A chair unsuited to a child will quickly induce special and bad habits of sitting and of breathing. In urbanized and industrialized communities bad habits in our motor acts are especially common. But verbal instruction as to how to correct wrong habits of movements and posture is very difficult. The scantiness of our sensory perception of how we do them makes it so. The faults tend to escape our direct observation and recognition. Of the proprioceptive reflexes as such, whether of muscles or ear (vestibule), we are unconscious. . . . Correcting the movements carried out by our proprioceptive reflexes is something like trying to reset a machine, whose works are intangible, and the net output all we know of the running. Instruction in such an act has to fall back on other factors more accessible to sense; thus, in skating, to 'feeling' that edge of the skate-blade on which the movement bears. To watch another performer trying the movement can be helpful; or a looking-glass in which to watch ourselves trying it. The mirror can tell us often more than can the most painstaking attempt to 'introspect'. Mr Alexander has done a service to the subject by insistently treating each act as involving the whole integrated individual, the whole psycho-physical man. To take a step is an affair, not of this or that limb solely, but of the total neuro-muscular activity of the moment—not least of the head and the neck.

"It is fortunate, my lord, as I have said, that the great Sir Charles Sherrington, before this case was started, has had occasion to make reference to the plaintiff, particularly when it is remembered that the plaintiff is branded in the present case as a charlatan. I think I should, in connection with the last passage I read from Sir Charles Sherrington's book, draw your lordship's attention to the fact that Sir Charles Sherrington had seen fit to quote, in a footnote, Mr Alexander's *Universal Constant in Living*.

"This brings me to the next step in outlining this technique. Mr Alexander, in his experiments on himself and in the teaching of teaching methods to others, had been led to observe the fact that in all misuses, all misuses of the body, there is a noticeable and prime misuse, more or less developed and present in all individuals who misuse themselves: namely, a tendency to tense the neck muscles in any activity; that if a man proceeds to lift something, or if he proceeds to get up from a chair, his prime misuse of himself is the tensing of the neck, evidenced in many cases by a tendency to pull the head and neck down in relation to the torso, that is, when the man gets up, sometimes imperceptibly, sometimes very noticeably. Look at the man who is rising out of a chair. It can be seen, in the effort to get up, that he tenses his neck and brings the head back and down, and, putting it rather shortly, perhaps over-simplifying it, that a correct head-neck relationship is a *sine qua non*, Mr Alexander discovered, to good posture. That, unless you can get a good head-neck relationship, faulty posture will result. That was proved by students of the Alexander Technique. They have the suspicion that you would have consequent misuses of the body in activity.

"Now, until such time as your lordship is invited to read the whole of *Man's Supreme Inheritance*, which is Mr Alexander's first work and therefore very important in this regard, I say that it abounds with illustrations of persons who came into Mr Alexander's rooms—of stutterers, stammerers and of persons who were brought there by doctors describing something about them—and in each case your lordship will see the observation that there was a tensing of the head and neck, or words which convey that. Mr Alexander, it must not be lost in this case, is no physiologist; he is no medical man; he is no scientific man. He was an elocutionist who was pursuing his methods by direct observation. He discovered, quite objectively, that if a man were taught to prevent this interference with a correct head-neck relationship, to prevent this tension of the head in activity, it had a marked effect on the whole mechanism, and to him the head-neck relationship was therefore of prime importance in its association with the functioning of the whole muscular mechanism of the man, and he wrote that if a man will *consciously prevent this tension of the head-neck in all his movements* he will not then interfere with the proper functioning of his whole mechanism. This can be achieved, as your lordship will gather, by a mental direction of 'head forward and up'. It does not mean that a man, a man who is using himself correctly, must move his head in space in relation to his body, but if he carries into practice the mental idea when performing an act, the mental conception, it will prevent the head being pulled down into the body and so giving rise to the tensing which Mr Alexander maintains affects the whole working of the body. And this is described in his two earlier works, *Man's Supreme Inheritance* and in *The Conscious Control of the Individual,* as the relationship of head-to-neck and head-to-neck to torso, or it is described as a position of mechanical advantage, which was a word used in those days to describe the most advantageous working position of the body, which always headed this particular relationship of the head and neck in which there was no tension.

"In 1932, when Mr Alexander produced a new work, that is *The Use of the Self,* he used the phrase 'primary control'. Your lordship, I hope, will be persuaded—I say persuaded because the defendant has introduced a lot of confusion about this—that he used the phrase 'primary control' to describe that self-same relationship he had always been talking about, namely the relationship of the head to the neck and the head and neck to the torso—'Primary', because it is first in time and first in importance; a phrase that has been used by great physiologists. I will endeavour to convey what that means.

"It means that the head moves and the body follows. The head is the prime directing force of the body in this relation. The head moves and the body follows. If the head moves correctly, the body will follow correctly; if the head moves incorrectly, the body will follow incorrectly. And this theory of 'conscious awareness', which is a philosophy of his earlier books on the destiny of man as applied to 'primary control', means this, that man must consciously not interfere with this relationship; he must consciously direct the head forward and up; he must consciously prevent it from tensing. Sir Charles Sherrington in the self same book has a short passage on this. It comes just a little before the passage I have read to your lordship a little while ago, but I omitted it because it would be meaningless until I had given this explanation. He writes: 'Today's knowledge teaches that every so-called "voluntary" muscle with its nervous supply is a little "reflex" system. Any act, of whatever provenance, which employs such a muscle cannot fail to enlist reflex action from it, and from muscles related to it—synergists, antagonists. These (proprioceptive) reflexes are unconscious as such, but on them depends in large part the rightness of the muscular act, and the possibility of physical perfection; it rests with each of us to attain it by personal understanding and effort.'

"Now, my lord, the libel gives very scanty reference to anything in the teachings of Mr Alexander that I have so far addressed your lordship on. To this I will revert again in a moment. But this point I prefer to make first, that some scathing references have been made to the fact that a world-famous philosopher, Professor John Dewey, has supported Mr Alexander. The scathing references are that it was puzzling to see that number of people, including Professor John Dewey, the philosopher, publicly praising 'the Australian actor'. On page 13 Professor John Dewey has scorn heaped upon him and is really described as being quite senile at the time that he supported Mr Alexander. It is stated there: 'Another admirer of Mr Alexander is Professor John Dewey, now aged 86, whose fame as a philosopher and educationalist is of course based on writings published when he was much younger. (His *Psychology* appeared in 1887; his *Study of Ethics* in 1894 and his last great work, *Human Nature and Conduct*, in 1922.)'

"The fact is that in *Human Nature and Conduct* Professor John Dewey produced a work which is described as one of his great works, and in it he devoted many pages to Mr Alexander. Some of them bear reading at this stage. The book, which will be proved in due course, contains many references between the pages of 68 and 134. I am not going to read all these pages, but this appears: 'Recently a friend remarked to me' [the friend, my lord, is Mr Alexander] 'that there was one superstition current amongst even cultivated persons. They suppose, *if* one is told what to do and if the right end is pointed to them, all that is required in order to bring about the right act is the will or wish on the part of the one who is to act.' He used as an illustration the matter of physical posture. The assumption is that if a man is told to stand up straight, all that is further needed is the wish and effort on his part and the deed is done. He pointed out that this belief is on a par with primitive magic in its neglect of attention to the means which are involved in reaching an end.

"He went on to say that the prevalence of his belief, starting with false notions about the control of the body and extending to the control of mind and character, is the greatest bar to intelligent social progress. It bars the way because it makes us neglect intelligent inquiry to discover the means which will produce the desired result, an intelligent invention to procure the means—in short it leaves out the importance of intelligent controlled habit. We may cite his illustration of the real nature of the physical act or order, its execution in contrast with the current false notion, and, I refer to Mr Alexander's *Man's Supreme Inheritance*.

A man who has had a bad habitual posture tells himself or is told to stand up straight. If he is interested and responds, he braces himself, goes through certain movements, and it is assumed that the desired result is substantially attained, that the position is retained at least as long as the man keeps the idea and order in his mind. Consider the assumptions that are here made. It is implied that the means or defective condition of the realization of the purpose exist independently of established habit and even that they may set in motion in opposition to habits. It is assumed that the means are there so that the failure to stand erect is wholly a matter of failure of purpose and desire. It needs paralysis or a broken leg or some other equally gross phenomenon to make us appreciate the importance of objective conditions. Now, in fact, a man who can stand properly does so, and only a man who can does. In the former case efforts of will are in the latter useless. A man who does not stand properly forms a habit of standing improperly, a positive forceful habit. The common implication that his mistake is merely negative and that he is simply failing to do the right thing and that the failure can be made good by a normal effort of will is absurd. One might as well suppose that the man who is the slave of whisky drinking is merely one who fails to drink water. Conditions have been formed for producing a bad result and the bad result will occur.

"Then, my lord, in the following pages, Professor John Dewey, who is a very famous American philosopher, actually incorporates Mr Alexander's teachings in his philosophy. It would take me too long at this stage, though it is only six pages, to read them to your lordship; reference will be made to them later. But there are two short passages to which I would like to refer: 'After we get to the point of recognizing that bad habits must intervene between wish and execution in the case of bodily acts, we still cherish the illusion that they can be dispensed with in the case of mental and moral acts. Thus the net result is to make a distinction between non-moral and moral activities, and lead us to confine the latter strictly within a private immaterial realm. But, in fact, formation of ideas as well as their execution depends on bodily habit . . .'

"And he then deals with his philosophy of mind and shows that moral and other purposes have also got something to do with the same basis of false habits. He concludes with this:

Our ideas truly depend upon experience, but so do our sensations, and the experience upon which they both depend is the operation of habits, originally of instincts. Thus our purposes and commands regarding action, whether physical or moral, come to us through the medium of bad bodily habits. The inability to think aright is sufficiently striking to have caught the attention of moralists but a false psychology has led them to interpret it as due to unnecessary conflict of flesh and spirit, not as an indication that our ideas are as dependent, to say the least, upon our bodily habits as are our acts upon our conscious thoughts and purposes.

"There are more passages, but I will not weary your lordship with them now. If Mr Alexander's ideas are sound, it would naturally follow that amongst persons who have practised his teaching there should have emerged illustrations of improvement in health. In fact, evidence will be put before your lordship to the effect that the application of this technique, its application in connection with the use of the human body, does improve posture, does improve the use of the individual. It will be proved to your lordship, through medical references, that bad posture has a serious effect upon good health, and that improvements in posture will benefit the whole organism. In order to teach this procedure, it requires patience, understanding and a power of application. Your lordship will also hear that many pupils fall by the way, because they have not got the powers to adapt themselves or to see it through.

"As in all progressive steps in human progress, the work is never confined to one man or to one place. Mr Alexander, acting quite independently, has evolved these theories, some of which may be optimistic, some of which may go a little far, but basically his lesson is that he has a method for teaching good use of the body and that is to improve health. It is not without significance that in other parts of the world, quite independently from Mr Alexander, similar work on similar thought has been taking place. In America in recent years, there has been a new development in the field of medicine, which has recently been called psychosomatic medicine, which is a more dignified way of putting Mr Alexander's psycho-physical. Evidence will be given to your lordship that reputable orthopaedic work in America is advancing along the lines that faulty body mechanics is at the root of much ill-health. It is perhaps fortunate that this action did not take place twenty years ago because the recent medical literature from America would not have been available for your lordship. It is fortunate that the informed and advancing medical opinion in these countries is now available to us in the form of recent works that will be proved in this case.

"In England, which apparently lags a little behind America in this, some medical support for Mr Alexander has been forthcoming over the years. Some 25 medical men over the years, from time to time, have been impressed with his methods and have written about them. Some of the younger people in England, who have been convinced of the basic soundness of his ideas, are present in this court today. They have come from England and your lordship will hear some of them in evidence; others have given evidence on commission in England. And I would also point to the fact that at the same time some confirmatory work was done by the scientist Coghill, who is referred to in this article.

"He was an eminent professor of anatomy, whose special work was embryology. The whole of his conclusions in the field of embryology, so he wrote, confirm Alexander's work, so much so that an appreciation was written by Coghill in the introduction to *The Universal Constant in Living*. He writes:

The practice of F. Matthias Alexander in treating the human body is founded, as I understand it, on three well-established biological principles: (1) that of the integration of the whole organism in the performance of particular functions; (2) that of proprioceptive sensitivity as a factor in determining posture; (3) that of the primary importance of posture in determining muscular action. These principles I have established through 40 years in anatomical and physiological study of Amblystoma in embryonic and larval stages, and they appear to hold for other vertebrates as well."

*   *   *

At this point the opening address went on to deal with the personal factors which had led to the writing of the defamatory article. Evidence which totalled more than 450,000 words was taken both in London and in Johannesburg and Alexander was awarded massive costs in addition to damages. Details of the judgement of the Supreme Court are given in Chapter 35.

FOUR

The Meaning of Misuse
by Dr Wilfred Barlow

MISUSE IS AN umbrella term for which no simple definition can be given. Alexander meant by "misuse" very much more than those distortions of the muscular and bony framework, which are the province of the orthopaedic surgeon, the physiotherapist, the osteopath and the physical educationist.

Firstly, misuse has to include the simple mechanical actions which we carry out all day and every day in moving ourselves and moving objects in our environment. I have detailed many of these in my book, *The Alexander Principle*—a good example is that of the pastry-cook (plate 1), who for twenty years has bent over a conveyer belt stamping out pastry. In the process he has developed a sideways curvature which persists even when he stops doing it, because the muscle tension involved in the work is not released. He has also (plate 2) developed an arthritic spur at the spot where he repeatedly presses down on his lumbar spine. Movement-misuse does not, however, result from vigorous activities only: more usually it arises in relation to quite simple movements of everyday life such as sitting and standing (plate 3) and it was around such movements that Alexander organized much of his re-educational work.

Secondly, misuse occurs in the various positionings and postures which we take up: sitting still, lying, standing, kneeling and all the variations of these. Over 1,000 such positions have been listed (*Scientific American* 196, 1957): very few of them require a misuse of the body—it is what goes on within these 1,000 different positions which matters: "it's not what you do, it's the way that you do it", as the popular song has it.

Thirdly, and perhaps more difficult to describe and to observe, are those forms of misuse which may occur when we communicate. In addition to the obvious ways of communicating by word and gesture, we most of us exhibit tiny signs which—unconsciously, automatically, and whether we like it or not—transmit a certain mood, quite contrary to our conscious intention. These signs may be hardly perceptible by ordinary conscious observation, but when we undertake a detailed re-education by Alexander's methods, we find that they are dependent on habitual patterns of muscular tension, which by their persistence and eventual irrelevance must be termed a "mis-use".

These tiny mood-signs, which Dewey called "Properties of sensitivity and delicate participative response", are part and parcel of our personal conscious life; they may, however, come to include unconscious fragments of some "rôle" which was of significance in the past but which is now irrelevant. Such small gestures, grimaces, mannerisms, and shifts of muscular tension will appear strange and inappropriate because their content and origin have been lost; they evoke from those around us reactions which we do not want and, as habits, may be far more difficult to eliminate than those already mentioned. It is significant that Alexander first described misuse in relation to communication, i.e. in his speaking habits; and it is only when we discover, as he did, a resting-state of muscle tension in which no "rôle" is expressed that we become aware of these irrelevant tensions.

Fourthly, we must also expect to see misuse in a large range of biological activities which are partly under voluntary and partly under involuntary control: such things as breathing, eating, excreting, and sex. The way in which we handle these needs or functions may bring the concept of misuse into the province of morals and social adjustment.

Misuse and Emotions
These various types of misuse do not of course occur independently; at any time we may see movement, posture, communication, and biological functioning intermingling in a composite muscular reaction, both emotional and behavioural. The manner of muscular use is especially bound up with the emotions, since muscle is not only the vehicle of speech and expressive gesture, but has at least a finger in a number of other emotional pies—for example, breathing regulation. And not only are emotional attitudes, say, of fear and aggression, mirrored immediately in the muscle, but also such moods as depression, excitement and evasion have their characteristic muscular patterns and postures. The Bible has it: "He that being often reproved, hardeneth his neck, shall be utterly condemned." This observation was not apparently confirmed by Freud who spoke enthusiastically of science being a "mighty power to stiffen one's neck in adversity!" Tegner's remarks were interesting in this connection: "Rigid, unbending religious principles may develop similarly unbending spines and muscles ... tension-pains are relatively common (and often quite intractable) in strict Baptists, Salvationists, Plymouth Brethren and so on."

This "attitude theory of emotion" stems from Darwin, who used the term "expressive action" to denote the movements, gestures and attitudes from which the existence of an underlying emotional state might be inferred—"such movements of expression reveal the thoughts of others more truly than do words, which may be falsified". Dr Robin Skynner, who had access to a group of my patients, found a close relationship between their habitual postural attitudes and their predominant psychological conflicts: "It also seemed clear that the release of specific tensions went parallel with the release and acceptance of attitudes and emotions of which they were not fully aware."

Behaviourally, it is clear that there can be no form of movement, posture, or communication which will not rely upon muscle for its manifestation. The hysteric in plate 4a has a repeated extension movement which Cameron (1947) described as "acting through or re-living a special circumscribed rôle with a constant theme ... with repetition it may become the preferred habitual mode of escape from conflict". Such "depersonalization" occurs as a result of muscular hypertension, in which postural awareness is diminished; the physiotherapist in plate 4b, who is doing a postural exercise, seems unlikely to improve her muscular awareness by behaving in this manner.

In time muscle is not only itself modified into recurrent patterns of misuse, but it modifies the bones and joints on which it works and the circulatory system which traverses it. As an anthropologist, Hooton (1936) put it: "The bony framework has been warped and cramped and stretched in one part or another in accordance with variations in the stresses and strains put upon it by different postures." It has sometimes been suggested by orthopaedic surgeons that repetitive movements do not produce lasting deformity, but this is clearly not the case. Plate 5 for example shows a young javelin thrower whose repeated movements have led to a sideways curvature: plate 6 shows a physical-training student who specialized in right-handed throwing activities. Her rotary twist at rest is apparent from the breast and arm position.

Alexander's concept of misuse is, however, more especially concerned with smaller persistent postures and gestures which gradually leave their mark on the organism until the resting state becomes deformed. "Man is not bent because he is old, but because his unconscious defences have bent him," was a view of Booth (1937) in a study of personality and chronic arthritis. Many people, indeed, will persist in a misuse even when it is producing pain. I have found it interesting in my out-patient clinics to ask patients who complain, say, of buttock-pain to describe to me the quality of their pain, whilst they lie relaxed, face downward on the bed. As they describe the quality of their pain, they almost always set up a state of muscular contraction in the painful buttock and even when they can be persuaded to release this muscular misuse, it will return when they think once more of their pain. Such "pain-making" by overtensing muscles is quite unconscious. Almost all misuse patterns are below the level of consciousness, and begin to influence the posture. Pain-making may occur in what might be called the "one fine day" syndrome, in which the patient, like Madame Butterfly, maintains a certain postural attitude, even though it is pain-producing, in order to be "right" for the departed loved one, against the day of possible return. We most of us tend to adopt the attitude of those we love— even in the cinema we may mimic in miniature those we identify with. Indeed, a family posture is often the expression of the basic family mood, e.g. the identical twins in plate 7. Rejection of the family mood may lead to rejection of the posture—"I can't stand like that, it feels just like the way my mother looks," as one girl with a chronic back pain said after her posture had been temporarily corrected.

Plate 8 is an interesting example of "pain-producing" by muscular fixation of the left shoulder. It can be seen that the muscle which runs from the left side of the neck down on to the top of the left shoulder is contracted so that the shoulder has been raised up. This particular person had in fact been discharged from the services because of pain in this area, although no one had noticed the "misuse" cause of the pain. This is another example of misuse which persists after certain behaviour because there is no knowledge of a proper resting state of balance.

It might also be appropriate here to mention the effect of carrying out forms of muscular exercise which involve over-contraction of muscle (see plate 9)—this is particularly harmful where there is already a structural deformity since not only will the deformity be increased but there is increasing inability to return to a balanced state of rest. The implications of this for physical education are tremendous.

In *The Alexander Principle*, I gave the example of a civil servant who had a severe arthritis of the neck with associated arm pain. It was possible to train him to release the tension which was deforming his neck, and in this position he was free from pain. Such, however, was his ingrained attitude of cringing in front of his superiors that he was unable to maintain the improved posture until he had eventually had a row with the boss. Such deforming attitudes of cringing and evasiveness eventually indeed will lead to structural change: for example the evasive action of perpetually turning the gaze away by turning the head to one side will often set up a persistent twist at the base of the neck.

Against this, Alexander has suggested, as did an orthopaedic surgeon, Goldthwaite, 1917, that "when the body is used rightly, all of the structures are in such adjustment that there is no strain on any part. The physical processes are at their best, the mental functions are performed most easily, and the personality or spirit of the individual possesses its greatest strength."

This is, however, easier said than done. Teenagers, who usually sit around in such slumped postures as figures 1c and 1d might feel "stuck up" if they were to sit up, using their bodies well, as in figure 1a, even if they misuse their knees, as in figure 1b. The value of conforming to the group pattern of slumping outweighs for them any other consideration. These conformity deformities are hard to avoid and it is difficult to be with a lot of other people who are "pulling down" without doing the same—all the more so when they are not aware that such habits are harmful.

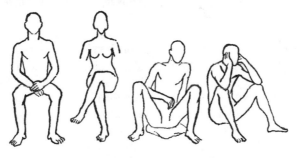

Figures 1a   1b   1c   1d

The Preferred Perception

It will be clear from what I have said that it is difficult to separate out the various components of misuse—the physiological, the emotional, the behavioural and the structural—in a given muscular reaction. A few years ago I suggested the term "postural homeostasis" to cover these comprehensive reactions of muscular self-regulation by which we adjust to our environment. A human being is not an amoeba, passively reacting on a stimulus-response basis within the limits of its biochemistry, but is constantly concerned with *the organization of a preferred perception*, whether it be the perception of a preferred personal body structure or the perception of a preferred set of external circumstances. Such an organization of perception is a motor act involving muscular use, and my purpose in introducing the term postural homeostasis was to imply that *after* activity, there should always be a return to a steady resting state. This concept is elaborated in chapter 8. Such a resting state can be described in anyone in terms of the preferred posture with its underlying pattern of preferred muscular tension. The resting state may be balanced or unbalanced, according to the degree of misuse. On this definition, misuse is the residual tension and postural deformity which remains after stress activity, as in plates 5 and 6. Indeed any activity which leaves a residual muscular tension is to that extent a stress activity. Such residual tension can either be resolved by returning to a balanced resting state, or it may be partially diminished without, however, the underlying tendency being resolved. In the latter case the tension pattern remains latent in an unbalanced resting state, so that it requires only the idea of the stress activity to reactivate the misuse, usually in the form of anticipatory tension or "set": and of course once the actual stress situation appears, there is a more obvious return to the habitual state of misuse, which is the muscular expression of the preferred way of perceiving it.

When one turns over the multitudinous complexities of muscular attitude and postural disposition, the possibility of a neat classification seems far off. Yet since the mind-body relationship is perhaps more clearly observable in muscular reactions than in any other postulated stress mechanism, the problem of classifying misuse cannot be insoluble and may ultimately illuminate the whole field of stress disorders, which are so difficult to treat.

Releasing Tension

The difficulty in re-educating tension patterns lies in the situation already described, that there are two ways of getting rid of undue tension. (1) The tension can be released or relaxed a little without the actual resolving of the underlying pattern of misuse, which remains latent until the conditions for its revival occur. (2) The tension can be resolved by a return to a balanced resting state, leaving no unconscious residue of misuse.

Owing to a lack of understanding of what is entailed by the balanced resting state of good use which Alexander described, most people, with or without the help of their doctor, resort to procedure (1). By avoiding the stress situation or the memory of it, the activation of the latent tension may be avoided, but this results in a lack of vitality, creativity, and enjoyment of forward planning (which would activate the tension state).

Why is it that Alexander's balanced resting state of good-use should be so difficult to attain? Firstly, there is widespread ignorance of what it entails. People simply do not know that they are misusing themselves in the way that the Alexander Principle indicates. Secondly, when someone is in a misused state, there is often a fear of a return to a state of proper muscular rest, since this would involve a realization of a "true" emotional experience, and the adjustment of the picture of reality. The preferred "body image" which we have of ourselves is usually sustained by organizing our muscular adjustment in a given way. By maintaining this faulty manner of use, it is possible to avoid knowledge of the discrepancy between the artificial picture we have of ourselves and the true picture which would become apparent in a balanced resting state of good use.

The Muscular Matrix of Decision

This clearly begins to take us a long way from a purely physical concept of misuse, into the sphere of values; and it was in this sphere that Alexander has seemed to many people to be his most mystifying. His concept of "the primary control" seemed not only to be saying that the muscular balance of our heads and necks had to be accurate if the rest of the body was to be well-used, but also that our conscious regulation of this primary head-neck balance in some way was to become the single most important control in our lives—that in some way full self-realization could depend on this factor which would supremely regulate all of our functions, and not simply be one balancing factor amongst many other balancing factors. He himself did not make it clear why the full expression of our nature should be so dependent upon our having such a single control which would apparently have such profound effects on our psychological functioning.

None of this has been adequately worked out—it seems to me—either in Alexander's writings or in what other people have written. Indeed since mind-body relationships have been a favourite topic with the philosophers for over 2,000 years, it would be rash to expect to avoid the traps and pitfalls. What I can see is that we must try to get away from any form of mind-body dualism—a dualism which states that there are two fundamental stuffs, quite different, which go to make up the human organism, and which must be approached and studied in an entirely different manner. Mind-body dualism permeates our present educational and medical institutions through and through, in spite of protestations to the contrary. In the educational world, the pupil is divided up and dealt with in at least two parts—a a mind which is to be taught in the classroom and a body which is to be taught on the playing field and in the gymnasium. In the medical world the departments of psychological medicine and general medicine tend to be very distinct entities.

The problem of mind-body dualism, however, goes far deeper than the medical and educational sides of it. Our entire social system demonstrates in its active working life this split between mind and body. The manual worker and the so-called brain worker fall into two definite class divisions and the body tends to get the worst of the bargain and to be placed lower down in the social hierarchy. Even more important than this social split is the actual effect which the two modes of life have on the worker, accentuating on the one hand the physical at the expense of the mental, and on the other hand the mental at the expense of the physical. The manual worker in field or factory is apt to become little more than an unthinking automaton. We may recall Charlie Chaplin's film, *Modern Times*, with the poor little man who works all day long at a conveyor belt, carrying out just one task, consisting in giving a twist with a spanner to a single bolt on each of the identical machines which stream past him. At the end of the day's work, Chaplin shows him outside the factory, still making these same twisting movements, unable to stop. His "resting state of balanced homeostasis" was indeed a long way off.

Yet who would say that the sedentary worker is any better off? Take a look at the typical morning tube train in London, with its load of office workers. Follow them to their office chairs where they sit in a dim unhealthy room, slumping down in a state of fatigue and boredom for much of the time. The sedentary worker is in danger of losing that minimum degree of activity which will enable him to maintain himself in a state fit for work. I have no wish to glorify the savage or natural state—salvation does not lie in a return to nature—but it is useful, I think, to remember that in the savage state, in the small integrated community, the urge for self-preservation took a man out into his surroundings to hunt or to cultivate the ground. Desire and execution were closely knit together in these men. They were as integrated with their environment as is the tennis player on the court, moving about freely to satisfy the next most obvious need. The sedentary worker is a far cry from all of this: his urge for self-preservation takes him into his office chair via a tube train, and often the chief interest that he has in his work is in his pay packet.

Alexander, as I have pointed out, does not seem to me to have adequately described just how it comes about that his "primary control" can be the single most important regent in our everyday affairs and enable us to regulate ourselves so that we can resolve this problem of mind-body dualism. What we can say is that we adopt a certain position or manner of use because, consciously or unconsciously, we consider it valuable. The first answer to the question "Why did I do that?" is always "Because I considered it valuable". If the reader would examine why he himself carries out his next action, he will have to answer it in this way—even if it only involves scratching his nose: that he scratches it because it seems valuable to him to scratch it. The next question is, of course "Why do I consider it valuable?", and to this the answers are individual and multitudinous. In the same way misuse patterns will seem valuable to us for us a multitude of reasons, some of them physiological, some of them psychological, some of them conscious, some of them unconscious. A laborious analysis of their antecedents has never been part of the Alexander Technique—it has been considered enough to re-train the faulty habit, since in the process of learning a new resting state of muscle balance, the pupil will eventually discover the values that lead him to destroy such a balance.

To speak of altering unconscious habits in such a manner will usually call down cries of "crude behaviourism" on one's head. Anyone who has been through the long drawn-out process of re-education which Alexander's work involves knows that there is nothing crude in this process. It is never a question of detecting a faulty habit pattern once and for all, de-conditioning it and seeing it disappear. Rather it is a matter of continually having to re-find it, in different situations. We fall into the same tricks of misuse again and again and the discovery of these tricks by no means stops us from repeating them.

We do, however, soon discover that, side by side with patterns of misuse, there is often an inability to stick to decisions, because constancy of decision seems to require constancy in the manner of use. With misuse, there is disintegration of intention—we find it hard to adhere to the mood in which we take a decision. This leads to avoidance of responsibility or of opportunity, or of procrastination in the face of jobs that are inevitable. Tasks are left unfinished, effort is disorganized and inadequate and there may be an inability to define sub-goals (means-whereby) which would lead to fulfilment of strong desires.

However, as misuse patterns begin to be reordered, there is a corresponding integration of intention: we begin to re-organize ourselves so as to cope with life more constructively, more intelligently and in a more adaptive way. We begin to change in our perception of ourselves and others, becoming less defensive and more tolerant of frustration. We begin to feel more alive, more buoyant; to experience an unexpected ease of functioning.

This connection between the physical and the psychological becomes clearer as an Alexander re-education proceeds. When, for example, we are misusing ourselves by "pulling down", we do not get the thoughts which would lead us out of the situation and which is depressing us. The remedy, at least in part, is to stop pulling down and wait for new ideas to arise: and arise they will when energy is not dissipated in misuse.

We are born to be free in our reactions, and this means the expression of freedom in our manner of use. Many people, however, prefer a deforming attitude of slavery to things and people. There is so often a persistent drag-down to a state of non-directing mediocrity in which increasing consciousness is feared because it would mean increasing awareness of truth. Those who have the courage to adopt a life-style of "good-use" begin to exhibit a greatly heightened vitality, not only physically but psychologically as well.

Conclusion

It is not easy when describing a procedure as novel as the Alexander Technique to strike a balance between the pretentious and the platitudinous. Yet it is inescapable that anyone, doctor or patient, who works at this technique will soon find himself involved in fundamental issues of decision. We most of us have, as part of our cultural heritage, an ethical notion that is normal and essential that the good should be difficult: "Hard work is what is good" (Pieper, 1952). And yet often it is the person who tries hardest to get rid of his habits of tension who generates the most tensions in the process. Certainly the chief need for the Alexander student is to cultivate an attentive resting state which is quite distinct from the state of slump and passive relaxation. If we are ever to have the "whole man", he will be the man who has mastered the art of attending to the here-and-now of his use in his everyday life.

APPLICATIONS

EDUCATIONAL

FIVE

A Psychophysical Education
by Aldous Huxley

IN THE WORLD as we know it, mind and body form a single organic whole. What happens in the mind affects the body; what happens in the body affects the mind. Education must therefore be a process of physical as well as mental training.

Of what nature should this physical training be? The question cannot be properly answered except in terms of our first principles. We are agreed that the ideal human being is one who is non-attached. It is difficult to find a single word that will adequately describe the ideal man of the free philosophers, the mystics, the founders of religions. "Non-attached" is perhaps the best. Accordingly all education, including physical education, must ultimately aim at producing non-attachment. If we would discover which is the best form of physical training, we must begin by setting forth the physical conditions of non-attachment.

First of all, it is pretty clear that non-attachment is very hardly realizable by anyone whose body is seriously maladjusted. A maladjusted body affects the mind in several ways. When the maladjustment is very great, the body is subject to pain and discomfort. Pain and discomfort invade the field of consciousness, with the result that the owner of the body finds great difficulty in not identifying himself with his faulty physical processes.

In other cases pain and discomfort may not be present; but the maladjusted body may be subject, without its owner being aware of the fact, to chronic strains and stresses. What happens in the body affects the mind. Physical strains set up psychological strains. The body is the instrument used by the mind to establish contact with the outside world. Any modification of this instrument must correspondingly modify the mind's relations with external reality. Where the body is maladjusted and under strain, the mind's relations, sensory, emotional, intellectual, conative, with external reality are likely to be unsatisfactory. And the same would seem to be true of the mind's relations with what may be called internal reality—with that more-than-self which, if we choose, we can discover within us and which the mystics have identified with God, the Law, the Light, the integrating principle of the world.

C

All the eastern mystics are insistent on the necessity of bodily health. A sick man cannot attain enlightenment. They further point out that it is very difficult for a man to acquire the art of contemplation unless he observes certain rules of diet and adopts certain bodily postures. Similar observations have been made by Christian mystics in the west. For example, the author of *The Cloud of Unknowing* insists that enlightenment, or mystical union with God, is unattainable by those who are physically uncontrolled to the extent of fidgeting, nervously laughing, making odd gestures and grimaces. Such tics and compulsions (it is a matter of observation) are almost invariably associated with physical maladjustment and strain. Where they exist, the highest forms of non-attachment are unachievable. It follows therefore that the ideal system of physical education must be one which relieves people of maladjustment and strain.

Another condition of non-attachment is awareness. Unawareness is one of the main sources of attachment or evil. "Forgive them, for they know not what they do." Those who know not what they do are indeed in need of forgiveness; for they are responsible for an immense amount of suffering. Yet more urgent than their need to be forgiven is their need to know. For if they knew, it may be that they would not perform those stupid and criminal acts whose ineluctable consequences no amount of human or divine forgiveness can prevent.

A good physical education should teach awareness on the physical plane—not the obsessive and unwished-for awareness that pain imposes upon the mind, but voluntary and intentional awareness. The body must be trained to think. True, this happens every time we learn a manual skill; our bodies think when we draw, or play golf, or take a piano lesson. But all such thinking is specialist thinking. What we need is an education for our bodies that shall be, on the bodily plane, liberal and not merely technical and narrowly specific. The awareness that our bodies need is the knowledge of some general principle of right integration, and along with it, a knowledge of the proper way to apply that principle in every phase of physical activity.

There can be no non-attachment without inhibition. When the state of non-attachment has become "a second nature", inhibition will doubtless no longer be necessary; for impulses requiring inhibition will not arise. Those in whom non-attachment is a permanent state are few. For everyone else, such impulses requiring inhibition arise with a distressing frequency. The technique of inhibition needs to be learnt on all the planes of our being. On the intellectual plane— for we cannot hope to think intelligently or to practise the simplest form of "recollection" unless we learn to inhibit irrelevant thoughts.

On the emotional plane—for we shall never reach even the lowest degree of non-attachment unless we can check as they arise the constant movements of malice and vanity, of lust and sloth, of avarice, anger and fear. On the physical plane—for if we are mal-adjusted (as most of us are in the circumstances of modern urban life), we cannot expect to achieve integration unless we inhibit our tendency to perform actions in the, to us, familiar, maladjusted way.

Mind and body are organically one; and it is therefore inherently likely that, if we can learn the art of conscious inhibition on the physical level, it will help us to acquire and practise the same art on the emotional and intellectual levels. What is needed is a practical morality working at every level from the bodily to the intellectual. A good physical education will be one which supplies the body with just such a practical morality. It will be a curative morality, a morality of inhibitions and conscious control, and at the same time, by promoting health and proper physical integration, it will be a system of what I have called preventive ethics, forestalling many kinds of trouble by never giving them the opportunity to arise.

So far as I am aware, the only system of physical education which fulfils all these conditions is the system developed by F. M. Alexander. Mr Alexander has given a full account of his system in his first three books, each of which is prefaced by Professor John Dewey. It is therefore unnecessary for me to describe it here—all the more so as no verbal description can do justice to a technique which involves the changing, by a long process of instruction on the part of the teacher and of active co-operation on that of the pupil, of an individual's sensory experiences. One cannot describe the experience of seeing the colour, red. Similarly one cannot describe the much more complex experience of improved physical co-ordination. A verbal description would mean something only to a person who had actually had the experience described; to the mal-co-ordinated person, the same words would mean something quite different. Inevitably, he would interpret them in terms of his own sensory experiences, which are those of a mal-co-ordinated person.

Complete understanding of the system can come only with the practice of it. All I need say in this place is that I am sure, as a matter of personal experience and observation, that it gives us all the things we have been looking for in a system of physical education: relief from strain due to maladjustment, and consequent improvement in physical and mental health; increased consciousness of the physical means employed to gain the ends proposed by the will, and, along with this, a general heightening of consciousness on all levels; a technique of inhibition, working on the physical level to prevent the body from slipping back, under the influence of greedy "end-gaining", into its old habits of mal-co-ordination, and working (by a kind of organic analogy) to inhibit undesirable impulses and irrelevance on the emotional and intellectual levels respectively.

We cannot ask more from any system of physical education; nor, if we seriously desire to alter human beings in a desirable direction, can we ask any less.

SIX

The Barrier of Habit
by John Dewey

(The American philosopher and educationist Professor John
Dewey, who died in 1952 at the age of 92, first met F. M.
Alexander at the time of the first world war and was deeply
impressed by the practical benefits and scientific soundness of his
teaching. Not only did Dewey write introductions to Alexander's
first three books, but he readily acknowledged that he owed the
concrete form of certain of his ideas to his experience of the
technique. In the following extract from *Human Nature and
Conduct* (1921), reproduced here by kind permission of Henry
Holt & Co., New York, Dewey discusses the implications of
Alexander's views on habit and will.)

F. M. ALEXANDER recently remarked to me that there was one
superstition current among even cultivated persons. They suppose
that if one is told what to do, if the right end is pointed out to them,
all that is required in order to bring about the right act is will or wish
on the part of the one who is to act.

He used as an illustration, the matter of physical posture; the
assumption is that if a man is told to stand up straight, all that is
further needed is wish and effort on his part, and the deed is done.
He pointed out that this belief is on a par with primitive magic in its
neglect of attention to the means which are involved in reaching an
end. He went on to say that the prevalence of this belief, starting with
false notions about the control of the body and extending to control
of mind and character, is the greatest bar to intelligent social progress.
It bars the way because it makes us neglect intelligent inquiry to
discover the means which will produce a desired result, and intelligent
invention to procure the means. In short, it leaves out the importance
of intelligently controlled habit.

We may cite his illustration of the real nature of a physical aim or
order and its execution in its contrast with the current false notion.
A man who has a bad habitual posture tells himself, or is told,
to stand up straight. If he is interested and responds, he braces
himself, goes through certain movements, and it is assumed that
the desired result is substantially attained; and that the position is

retained at least as long as the man keeps the idea or order in his mind.

Consider the assumptions which are here made. It is implied that the means or effective conditions of the realization of a purpose exist independently of established habit and even that they may be set in motion in opposition to habit. It is assumed that means are there, so that the failure to stand erect is wholly a matter of failure of purpose and desire. It needs paralysis or a broken leg or some other equally gross phenomenon to make us appreciate the importance of objective conditions. . . .

Conditions have been formed for producing a bad result, and the bad result will occur as long as those conditions exist. They can no more be dismissed by a direct effort of will than the conditions which create drought can be dispelled by whistling for wind. It is as reasonable to expect a fire to go out when it is ordered to stop burning as to suppose that a man can stand straight in consequence of a direct action of thought and desire. The fire can be put out only by changing objective conditions; it is the same with rectification of bad posture.

Of course, something happens when a man acts upon his idea of standing straight. For a little while, he stands differently, but only a different kind of badly. He then takes the unaccustomed feeling which accompanies his unusual stance as evidence that he is now standing right. But there are many ways of standing badly, and he has simply shifted his usual way to a compensatory bad way at some opposite extreme.

When we realize that fact, we are likely to suppose that it exists because control of the *body* is physical and hence is external to mind and will. Transfer the command inside character and mind, and it is fancied that an idea of an end and the desire to realize it will take immediate effect. After we get to the point of recognizing that habits must intervene between wish and execution in the case of bodily acts, we still cherish the illusion that they can be dispensed with in the case of mental and moral acts. Thus the net result is to make us sharpen the distinction between non-moral and moral activities, and to lead us to confine the latter strictly within a private, immaterial realm.

But in fact, formation of ideas as well as their execution depends upon habit. *If* we could form a correct idea without a correct habit, then possibly we could carry it out irrespective of habit. But a wish gets definite form only in connection with an idea, and an idea gets shape and consistency only when it has a habit back of it. Only when a man can already perform an act of standing straight does he know what it is like to have a right posture and only then can he summon the idea required for proper execution. The act must come before the thought, and a habit before an ability to evoke the thought at will. Ordinary psychology reverses the actual state of affairs.

Ideas, thoughts of ends, are not spontaneously generated. There is no immaculate conception of meanings or purposes. Reason pure of all influence from prior habit is a fiction. But pure sensations out of which ideas can be framed apart from habit are equally fictitious. The sensations and ideas which are the "stuff" of thought and purpose are alike affected by habits manifested in the acts which give rise to sensations and meanings. . . .

Admission that the idea of, say, standing erect is dependent upon sensory materials is, therefore, equivalent to recognition that it is dependent upon the habitual attitudes which govern concrete sensory materials. The medium of habit filters all the material that reaches our perception and thought. The filter is not, however, chemically pure. It is a reagent which adds new qualities and re-arranges what is received. Our ideas truly depend upon experience, but so do our sensations. And the experience upon which they both depend is the operation of habits—originally of instincts. Thus our purposes and commands regarding action (whether physical or moral) come to us through the refracting medium of bodily and moral habits. . . .

What is true of the dependence of execution of an idea upon habit is true, then, of the formation and quality of the idea. Suppose that by a happy chance a right concrete idea or purpose—concrete, not simply correct in words—has been hit upon: What happens when one with an incorrect habit tries to act in accord with it? Clearly the idea can be carried into execution only with a mechanism already there. If this is defective or perverted, the best intention in the world will yield bad results. In the case of no other engine does one suppose that a defective machine will turn out goods simply because it is invited to. Everywhere else we recognize that the design and structure of the agency employed tell directly upon the work done.

Given a bad habit and the "will" or mental direction to get a good result, and the actual happening is a reverse or looking-glass manifestation of the usual fault—compensatory twist in the opposite direction. Refusal to recognize this fact only leads to a separation of mind from body, and to supposing that mental or "psychical" mechanisms are different in kind from those of bodily operations and independent of them. So deep-seated is this notion that even so "scientific" a theory as modern psychoanalysis thinks that mental habits can be straightened out by some kind of purely psychical manipulation without reference to the distortions of sensation and perception which are due to bad bodily sets. The other side of the error is found in the notion of "scientific" nerve physiologists that it is only necessary to locate a particular diseased cell or local lesion, independent of the whole complex of organic habits, in order to rectify conduct.

Means are means; they are intermediates, middle terms. To grasp this fact is to have done with the ordinary dualism of means and ends. The "end" is merely a series of acts viewed at a remote stage; and a means is merely the series viewed at an earlier one. The distinction of means and end arises in surveying the *course* of a proposed *line* of action, a connected series in time. The "end" is the last act thought of; the means are the acts to be performed prior to it in time. To *reach* an end we must take our mind off from it and attend to the act which is next to be performed. We must make that the end. The only exception to this statement is in cases where customary habit determines the course of the series. Then all that is wanted is a cue to set it off. But when the proposed end involves any deviation from usual action, or any rectification of it—as in the case of standing straight—then the main thing is to find some act which is different from the usual one.

The discovery and performance of this unaccustomed act is the "end" to which we must devote all attention. Otherwise we shall simply do the old thing over again, no matter what is our conscious command. The only way of accomplishing this discovery is through a flank movement. We must stop even thinking of standing up straight. To think of it is fatal, for it commits us to the operation of an established habit of standing wrong. We must find an act within our power which is disconnected from any thought about standing. We must start to do another thing which on one side inhibits our falling into the customary bad position and on the other side is the beginning of a series of acts which may lead into the correct posture. The technique of this process is stated in Alexander's book, *Man's Supreme Inheritance*, and the theoretical statement given is borrowed from Mr Alexander's analysis.

The hard drinker who keeps thinking of not drinking is doing what he can to initiate the acts which lead to drinking. He is starting with the stimulus to this habit. To succeed he must find some positive interest or line of action which will inhibit the drinking series and which by instituting another course of action will bring him to his desired end. In short, the man's true aim is to discover some course of action, having nothing to do with the habit of drink or standing erect, which will take him where he wants to go. The discovery of this other series is at once his means and his end. Until one takes intermediate acts seriously enough to treat them as ends, one wastes one's time in any effort at change of habits. Of the intermediate acts, the most important is the *next* one. The first or earliest means is the most important *end* to discover.

SEVEN

The F. Matthias Alexander Technique and its Relation to Education
by I. G. Griffith

(An excerpt from an address delivered to the annual
conference of the Transvaal Teachers' Association)

MAN HAS CEASED to be a natural animal. Everything connected
with his life has changed—his environment, his food, his manner of
living—all have changed. No longer is he dependent on his physical
organism for his means of subsistence. Even where, to some extent,
he still depends on his physical organism, as in agriculture and some
trades, his muscles are being used in new ways, mainly in mechanical
repetitions of the same act. His habits have changed, but he himself,
as an entity, has not kept pace with the changes.

The last century has seen the greatest advance of all in man's
transition from the savage to the civilized stage in the introduction of
machinery to the point where man has conquered the land, the sea,
and the air, and, in doing so, has even conquered himself, in that he
has failed to keep pace in his own development. In fact a degeneration
has taken place. That this has been recognized is clear in the many
attempts made, even in our time, to instil into men's minds the
"back-to-nature" idea. These have been definite efforts to make man
a more natural being than he has become through the centuries of
development from the savage state, culminating in this era of scientific
achievement in which we live. This is also an era which has necessi-
tated the appearance of the psychologist and the psychiatrist, who
must endeavour to help man to undo so much of what he has done to
himself and to enable him to understand himself. In brief, man's
adaptability to the changes he himself has introduced has not kept
pace with those changes.

Still clearer proof of the recognition of the unsatisfactory state of
man in his mental, nervous, and muscular debility can be seen in the
remedies designed to bring about improvement. Among the best
known are physical culture, deep breathing, and relaxation.

Physical culture may be described as the attempt to remedy the
ills arising from artificial conditions. Bodily defects must result from

the disuse and misuse of muscles and energy formerly employed in the natural state to provide a means of livelihood. The remedy is to exercise these muscles and energies for given periods every day in the hope that they will be restored to their natural functions. You have no doubt tried this and given it up. There is no co-ordination, with resulting conflict and strife. Some benefits do accrue if the exercises are persisted in, but sooner or later, according to Alexander, other defects must gradually develop which finally outweigh whatever good originally resulted.

Deep breathing is a development from the physical-culture idea. It is the recognition that strenuous exercise may result in new and greater evils than those previously existing. Deep breathing, however, does not go to the root of the matter, which is the eradication of defects. This fact has been recognized by the compilers of the *Syllabus for Physical Education.* In that book occurs the following passage: "No mention is made in this syllabus of what is known as breathing exercises. In Ling's gymnastics, breathing exercises were given a fixed place in the gymnastic lesson. In the light of the latest physiological researches, however, this has been proved wrong."

Relaxation also failed. Practically every person when instructed or asked to relax collapses—that is, there is a general relaxation of muscles, the fact being ignored that many muscles were intended by nature to be tensed and others were intended to be more or less relaxed. If relaxation is persisted in there follows a lowering of vitality which is felt when regular duties are taken up again, and the old troubles reappear in a worse form.

The reason for the one-sidedness of these views has been the general acceptance of the idea that man is body, mind, and soul. More generally, the human being is classified as consisting of two parts—body and mind. Undoubtedly, in his original state man was a combination of both, a unity. Both aspects of his life worked together —in other words, they were co-ordinated. During his transition from savagery to civilization, man's use and development of the so-called mental side proceeded proportionately at a much greater rate than his use and development of the so-called physical side. As new forms of life developed there was relatively less demand on the so-called physical and more on the so-called mental side. This resulted in a lessening in the co-ordination between the two, which reached its peak in this present age, which we ourselves describe as a "complex life". This false distinction between body and mind is almost universal, and is an idea which must be rejected, so that we recognize man not as a being with two sides, physical and mental, but as a complete entity—a psychophysical organism. This is a conception which requires recognition in practice by educationists more than anyone else, so that we cease to consider our task to be the development of the child's mental side, and realize instead that we are concerned not with the mental aspect and the physical aspect separately, but with a psychophysical organism.

How, then, is this co-ordination to be achieved? How is the deterioration in the so-called physical side to be arrested and an improvement brought about? The deterioration has taken place mainly in our manner of use of ourselves in those habitual movements and actions which are subconsciously controlled, the way in which we use ourselves when we sit, stand, walk, and speak, for example. Subconscious control is failing us. To improve the position we must turn to a conscious control of our manner of use. This does not mean the specific control which we usually conceive of when we wish to move a muscle voluntarily, but implies the value and use of a conscious guidance and control applied constantly in all spheres where the psychophysical organism is concerned. Conscious control is dependent, first and foremost, upon the prevention of wrong habits of use, what Alexander calls inhibition, and second, upon the realization and understanding of the methods or means-whereby by which an improvement may be brought about.

To illustrate this conception, I wish to refer to the manner-of-use employed by children when writing. We are all familiar with the bent backs, twisted bodies and legs, excruciatingly bent fingers, and eyes too near to the books which are to be seen in the great majority of children when they set about the business of writing. None of us like this. A few try to improve the positions of the children, realizing that a manner of use such as this can be nothing but harmful. Watch your class when next you give the order to write, and you will see a clear example of end-gaining. The child's object or end is to write, and immediately each one literally grabs a pen and begins, inevitably adopting that wrong manner of use which all of us will admit is harmful. Why does this wrong manner of use persist? Because no child ever stops to think of the means whereby the act of writing should be performed. He has never been taught to think about it, and, in his endeavour to end-gain, has adopted any means-whereby, in practically every case, a wrong one. You cannot change that manner of use by saying, "Do this instead of that," because the same habitual use will take place in an endeavour to end-gain. The manner of use is wrong. End-gaining comes before the means-whereby. This conception is very fully examined and explained by F. M. Alexander in his book *The Universal Constant in Living*, in which he discusses the means-whereby necessary to bring about an improvement. The first condition is that of withholding action, of non-doing—that is, to refuse to end-gain. To achieve this, however, we fail if we employ a *direct* means-whereby. Alexander emphasizes that to prevent misdirection an *indirect* means-whereby must be employed.

"Non-doing," says Alexander, "is not a form of passivity, but an act of inhibition which comes into play when we refuse to give consent to certain activity in response to a given stimulus and thus prevent ourselves from sending those messages which would ordinarily bring about the habitual reaction resulting in the doing within the self of what we no longer wish to do." We have to learn that on receipt of a stimulus to activity, we must make a decision not to give consent to do anything in response, for this "doing" would simply mean the projection of the habitual responses which result in a wrong manner of use. If the old messages are inhibited, the old response will not be used, and it is then possible to substitute a new means-whereby for the carrying out of the action. This is the meaning and implication of inhibition.

If anything is done wrongly by children, the chief means employed by teachers to put it right is to tell them what to do instead. Thus, to improve the writing position, children are told to hold the pen in a certain way and to sit in a certain way. Now, the one thing that *is* certain is that the children will not use the right way told them by the teacher, because that right way will feel wrong. After all, people never do what they feel to be wrong when they are trying to be right. Furthermore, every child interprets the instructions given to him in terms of his own personal sensory experience. That experience is naturally different in every child.

The most obvious and common way in which man has failed to adapt himself to changing conditions is in this matter of sensory experience. Our sensory appreciation has become unreliable. This is easily seen, for you, as teachers, will know how often a child, when told to do a certain thing, will do it incorrectly. You will find this most common in actions which have to be performed with the hands—the method of holding a pen, for example. The teacher explains and demonstrates, and yet most of the children do a simple thing wrongly, to the great exasperation and irritation of the teacher. Are such children deliberately doing it wrongly? Surely not, for remember, people never do what they *feel* to be wrong when they are trying to be right. This is the point teachers must realize: those children *think* they are doing what they were told to do, and they feel they are doing it in the right way. Their sensory appreciation is at fault. I have asked many adults to do such an apparently simple thing as to put the head forward and up. Not one I have asked has been able to do it, but almost every one of them actually put the head back. All of them considered they had done what they had been asked to do, and to them it *felt* as if they had done the correct thing. This unreliable sensory appreciation results in our acceptance of certain ways of doing things because they *feel* right, and they feel right because we have always done them in those ways. An adult expressed his opinion to me very firmly that the natural way for a book in which one is writing to be placed is for it to be inclined to the left of the body at an angle of more than 45 degrees. He maintained this because it felt right to him, and it felt right because he had always placed his book in that way.

Two facts of great importance arise from this. The first is the universal confusion between the habitual and the natural or right way. So many people persist in saying that a manner of doing something is natural because for them it has become the habitual manner, and because it is habitual it is, therefore, right—an argument which, of course, will not hold water. The other fact is that it is impossible to do a thing in the right way when it has always been done in the wrong way, because the right way has never been experienced. One must actually feel or experience the right way before one can perform it or even recognize that the old way is wrong. "Do as you are told" is a command frequently on teachers' lips. The child holds his pen wrongly, and the teacher insists that he hold it as he was told to do. How can he, until he has *experienced*, not merely heard, how to do it? How can he, until he learns to inhibit the habitual response to the command, until he learns to stop "doing" and to think of the means-whereby? I can think of nothing more important for teachers to realize and appreciate than these facts, (*a*) that sensory experience is unreliable, and (*b*) that we cannot do a thing in the right way until we have actually experienced that right way.

What, then, can teachers do? Not very much until they know more about the matter of manner of use and its constant influence for good or ill, until they have some practical experience of inhibition—and the substitution of means-whereby for end-gaining—and of the part played by the primary control. Here it is necessary to say that the Alexander technique cannot be properly understood and its implications fully realized merely by listening to a talk or by reading Alexander's books. You must experience at least this much, your own wrong manner of use, your own unreliable sensory appreciation, and your own tendency to end-gain. This much is possible for those who are sufficiently interested to acquire some preliminary knowledge of the principles underlying the Technique, for they can be given a practical demonstration on themselves which will make the meaning of these three things I have just mentioned much clearer.

Man, know thyself. You cannot take out the mote from your brother's eye until you have first removed the beam from your own eye. It behoves us, therefore, to know ourselves, our own defects and failings, our own bad manner of use, and the consequent influence for ill on all our functioning; to know how to bring about an improvement in ourselves. Knowing ourselves, we shall find it necessary for us to learn to know the children we deal with—not to know them in the way we usually mean, but to know them as we ought to know ourselves. Then will come understanding of the working of the psychophysical organism, and with that understanding will come the will and ability to help these children that they may live more abundantly.

EIGHT

Physical Education Research
by Dr Wilfred Barlow

INTRODUCTION

A MAJOR THEME of Alexander's writing was the inadequacy of physical education in schools. The idea that physical fitness could be achieved by brief periods of physical exercise made no sense to him, since he had a vision of a way of life in which the body was to be used well and actively during even the most sedentary of pursuits. It is suprising though that so little has been done to incorporate his teaching into physical education programmes, and it is even more suprising that athletes and sportsmen generally have not taken more notice of the help that the Alexander Technique can offer. The injury-proneness of certain sportsmen seems to be clearly linked with their persistent misuse, and someone with an Alexander-trained eye can often see the deterioration in performance which goes hand in hand with the deterioration of the use of the body. Indeed it is usually only the sportsmen with, say, back pain or tendon trouble or perhaps breathing difficulties who find their way to an Alexander teacher, whereas another contribution lies in the achieving of peak condition and the prevention of injury. One of my own major motivations in taking up Alexander's work lay in the recurrent dislocation of one of my shoulders—a dislocation originally done playing football and perpetuated by accidents when skiing, diving, and playing ball-games. My disability was so great that I played in the Eton Fives match for Oxford against Cambridge—which incidentally we won—with my left arm strapped to my side. Nevertheless, it was not until Alexander had shown me how my arms and shoulders should be used properly that I was able once and for all to get rid of artificial restriction and to take part in many sporting activities without fear.

My medical bias has never made it possible for me to extend my research far into the field of physical education, but the following papers were a beginning. It is interesting that at first I was refused permission to publish the paper "An Investigation into Kinaesthesia" —it was written during the second world war and I was informed that it would be "prejudicial to army morale" if I showed that our young army cadets had anything the matter with them. When the war against Hitler was won, I was allowed to publish it, and I still treasure the correspondence—a masterpiece of bumbledom. Incidentally the research which I carried out in the army was viewed with tolerant amusement by those I served with—"Heads up, men" the sergeant-major would cry as I passed by, and to a man a platoon of soldiers would stiffen their necks and retract their skulls even further backwards and downwards, in blind obedience: theirs not to reason why, and I confess to shirking the major task, as a very young regimental medical officer, of pointing out the error of their ways, except by writing about it.

The first paper is also interesting in that I asked Alexander to define what he meant by kinaesthesia. We worked together at such a definition for a very long time, in the attempt to bring out clearly the psycho-physical implications of the term. The result is still not very satisfactory.

The second piece came about as a result of a bet. I had already carried out a study at The Royal College of Music (chapter 22) to see the effect of Alexander training on musicians. I was at that time carrying on a running battle with Gwynneth Thurburn, the Principal of Central School, to try to persuade her that her voice-training methods were wrong in many respects. Grudgingly—she is now the oldest of old friends and will confirm what I say—she conceded point by point where Alexander was right. Since she was, and is, a woman of very strong personality, she thereupon insisted that a large number of her staff should take Alexander instruction. From this Clifford Turner, the voice teacher at RADA, became interested, and from this, via John Fernald and Hugh Cruttwell, the present dominant position of the Alexander Technique in the drama world was established. Gwynneth Thurburn accepted my challenge that we should have an external observer (Professor J. M. Tanner) who would carefully measure after twelve months the "USE" of (a) a group of Alexander-trained students and (b) a group of Central-trained students, having of course measured them before they started. The results showed clearly that the Alexander group had improved markedly, whilst the Central group had deteriorated. But, most important, we had now shown that we had a method for reliably improving the manner of use, and once this fact was established, the effect of such a method could then be ascertained in whatever medical or educational situations we might like to try it out.

I   AN INVESTIGATION INTO KINAESTHESIA
by Wilfred Barlow, Captain, RAMC

Introduction
In recent years considerable claims have been put forward about the
work of a layman, Mr F. M. Alexander, and it is said that he has made
an important biological discovery which throws light on the problem
of the maintenance of health under conditions of modern civilization.
He has written several books on his work, setting out his thesis,
and he has received support from various sources: doctors, scientists,
teachers, politicians and religious leaders have testified that has he
certainly made a very important discovery. In recent years the weight
of medical support for his teaching has grown, and in 1937 the
British Medical Journal (page 1137) contained a letter from a group
of nineteen doctors, urging that "as soon as possible, steps be taken
for an investigation of Alexander's work".

The Nature of the Present Investigation
The present investigation was concerned with one of Alexander's
fundamental premises, which deals with the unreliability of certain
aspects of the kinaesthesia upon which people base the control and
direction of their bodily activities. The term "kinaesthesia" is taken
in this discussion to mean "The awareness which we have of our
manner of using our muscular mechanisms, at rest and in motion".
It is taken to include the sensory awareness which allows our activities
to be integrated into a total response—the sense by which we gauge
the amount of muscular tension which needs to be exerted in carrying
out our activities. It is also taken to include the beliefs which we have
about our muscular capabilities—the habitual pattern of sensory
awareness which gives or denies us confidence in carrying out our
muscular activities. Kinaesthesia cannot be studied satisfactorily
without taking into account the pattern of assessment and belief
which underlies it, i.e., the psychophysical correlation.

The investigation was carried out on two groups of army cadets,
between the ages of 17 and 22. These men were fairly representative
of their age groups in the general population, passed as fit by army
standards and as potential officers they could be expected to co-operate
intelligently in the investigation.

An Outline of Alexander's Theory
Before describing the observations, it will be necessary to touch on

certain aspects of Alexander's teaching. In his book, *The Use of the Self*, Alexander states: "Instinctive control and direction of Use has become so unsatisfactory, and the associated feeling so untrustworthy a guide, that it can lead us to do the very opposite of what we wish to do, or think we are doing." Again, he states: "The deceptiveness of the impressions which we get through our kinaesthesia, reaches such a pitch that these impressions can mislead us into believing that we are doing something with some part of ourselves when actually we can be proved to be doing something quite different." A little elaboration will make it clear what he means by this.

Alexander claims that under present conditions of civilization it is a matter of direct observation that we are nearly all of us misusing ourselves in our daily activities, failing to use ourselves mechanically to the best advantage as we maintain ourselves in posture and in activity. Moreover, the majority of people are not aware that they are misusing themselves, and, in fact, their misuse feels right and comfortable to them. Under civilized conditions, says Alexander, there has been a breakdown in the purely *instinctive* control and direction of the mechanical use of the body. Modern man is subjected to widely varying and quickly changing conditions of life, conditions very different from those met with in pre-civilized times: on the one hand there is a demand for static and sedentary modes of living: on the other, there is a demand for feats of complicated manipulation and movement and co-ordination; for example, the driving of a car or a tractor, or even the hitting of a golf ball. Instinctive (by which is meant habitual, unthinking, automatic) control and management of the mechanical use of the body, though it may have served man well in the savage state, has not proved adequate in our modern urban civilization, and, indeed, reliance upon it has led to a widespread deterioration in the co-ordinated use of the body.

These considerations led Alexander to a study of the control and direction of the muscular mechanisms, and particularly of the *sensory background* which constitutes the conception of the rightness or wrongness of the act performed. Sherrington, in his book, *Man on His Nature* (p. 174), stated the quandary in which man finds himself when he comes to consider the way in which he uses his muscular mechanisms, when he wrote:

Take this act of *standing*. Suppose my mind's attention be drawn to it, then I become fully aware that I stand. It seems to me an act fairly simple to do. I remember, however, that it cannot be very simple. That to execute it must require among other things the right degree of action of a great many muscles and nerves, some hundreds of thousands of nerve fibres, and of perhaps a hundred times as many muscle fibres. I reflect that various parts of my brain are involved in the co-ordinative management of all this, and that in doing so, my brain's rightness of action rests on receiving and despatching thousands of nerve messages, registering and adjusting pressure, tensions, etc., in various parts of me. Remembering this, I am perhaps rather disappointed at the very little my mind has to tell me about my standing.

Alexander was led to inquire in detail into what "my mind has to tell me about my standing", and also into what it had to tell him about the way he used himself in other co-ordinated activities. He came to the conclusion that not only does the "mind" tell us very little about the way we are using our muscular mechanisms, but that the very little which it does tell us is frequently not accurate: our awareness of activity is often so defective and unreliable that "it can lead us to do the very opposite of what we wish to do or think we are doing".

It is Alexander's claim, then, that there has occurred a widespread deterioration in the use of the muscular mechanisms of the body, and that this deterioration is accompanied by a deterioration in the sensory awareness of the misuse, so that the misuse can feel right and comfortable when it is in actual fact exerting a harmful effect on bodily functioning, and preventing maximum efficiency.

The Observations

According to Alexander, the misuse of the muscular mechanisms is especially shown by the movement of the head in space, relative to the neck and trunk, during activity.

> If you ask someone to *sit down*, you will observe, if you watch their actions closely, that in nearly all cases there is an undue increase of muscular tension in the body and lower limbs: in many cases the arms are actually employed. As a rule, however, the most striking action is *the alteration in the position of the head*, which is thrown back, whilst the neck is stiffened and shortened. (*Man's Supreme Inheritance*, p. 283.)

This is clearly a matter of simple observation, and as such should be verifiable without difficulty. The purpose of the present observations was to combine two things: firstly, to observe whether the head is in fact usually thrown back when the subject carries out the activity of sitting down, and secondly, to ascertain the extent of the subject's awareness of this manner of use of the head-neck relationship—to ascertain whether the subject knows what he is doing with himself, and whether what he thinks he is doing with himself corresponds with what he can be shown to be doing in practice.

The subjects were requested to stand in front of a chair in the usual standing position, and a light tape-measure was fixed with tape to hang freely downwards from the occipital protuberance, exerting a minimal tension on the back of the head, but hanging freely under its own weight (see Figs. 2 and 3). A horizontal line was drawn over

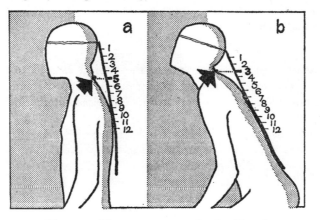

Figure 2. Tape measure on back of head

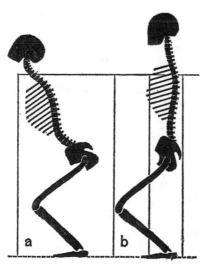

Figure 3. *a.* Head retraction in sitting down. *b.* Good use in sitting down

the 7th cervical spinous process with a skin-marking pencil. It was now possible by watching the tape-measure to assess the relationship of the occipital protuberance to the 7th cervical spinous process during the simple activity of sitting down, an activity which lends itself readily to observation. The observed relationship between the occipital protuberance and the 7th cervical spinous process has been termed the O-C (occipito-cervical) approximation in the account which follows.

In the first group of 56 cadets examined, 41 were aged 18, nine aged 19, three aged 21, and three aged 22 years. The results have been consolidated below.

Observation 1 In this observation, the subject is told to sit down twice in his customary manner, whilst the O-C approximation is read off, the point of maximum approximation being noted. The mean of two readings is given below.

O-C approximation	*No.*
No approximation	0
$\frac{1}{2}$ inch and under	4
1 inch—$\frac{1}{2}$ inch	7
2 inches—1 inch	35
Over 2 inches	10

It will be seen that in the majority of cases there was a considerable alteration in the position of the head, which was thrown back. None of the subjects were aware of the nature of the observation.

Observation 2 In this observation, the subject is asked if he has been aware of approximation occurring in Observation 1.

Aware of approximation	3
Unaware of approximation	53

These answers are not of great value in themselves, since the attention of the subject was not focused beforehand in the head-neck relationships: but as a result of the questioning, the way is paved for the next observation.

Observation 3 In this observation, the subject is again asked to sit down, but his attention has been focused on his head-neck relationship by the previous questioning.

O-C approximation	No.
No approximation	0
½ inch and under	8
1 inch—½ inch	11
2 inches—1 inch	33
Over 2 inches	4

In this observation, the subject is now "thinking about" his head-neck relationship because of the previous questioning.

Observation 4 In this observation, the subject is asked if he felt approximation occurring in Observation 3.

No. showing approximation	O-C approximation	No. who felt it	No. who did not feel it
8	½ inch and under	3	5
11	1 inch—½ inch	2	9
33	2 inches—1 inch	6	27
4	Over 2 inches	1	3

With their attention focused on it, 12 now said they could feel approximation occurring. The remainder could not feel it.

Observation 5 In this observation, the subject is requested consciously to prevent approximation occurring whilst he sits down: i.e., to do what he feels will prevent it occurring. All the subjects stated that they felt they were preventing approximation.

O-C approximation	No.
No approximation	7
½ inch and under	10
1 inch—½ inch	33
2 inches—1 inch	6
Over 2 inches	0

This is the clearest observation of all, for the subject is trying his best to prevent approximation, and "feels" he is preventing approximation. In spite of this, considerable approximation still occurs.

Taking observations 3, 4 and 5 together:

Observation 3		Observation 4		Observation 5 O-C approximation			
O-C approximation	No.	Feeling	Abs't	½" and under	1–½"	2–1"	Over 2"
½ inch and under	3	Yes	1	2	0	0	0
½ inch and under	5	No	2	2	1	0	0
1 inch—½ inch	2	Yes	0	0	2	0	0
1 inch—½ inch	9	No	2	2	5	0	0
2 inches—1 inch	6	Yes	0	0	5	1	0
2 inches—1 inch	27	No	2	4	18	3	0
Over 2 inches	1	Yes	0	0	0	1	0
Over 2 inches	3	No	0	0	2	1	0

These observations showed that:

1 Out of 56 cadets, all without exception showed a greater or less degree of O-C approximation when sitting down in their usual unthinking manner, and of these only three were aware of the approximation when their attention was first drawn to it.

2 Out of 56 cadets, only seven were able to prevent approximation when they tried.

3 Out of 56 cadets, 12 stated that they could feel approximation occurring after their attention had been drawn to it. Of these 12, only one could prevent approximation occurring when he tried: the remaining 11 considered that they were preventing approximation occurring when they were in actual fact approximating between ½ inch and 2 inches.

4 Out of 56 cadets, 44 said they could not feel approximation occurring when their attention was focused on it and when they were seen to be approximating. When asked consciously to prevent approximation, 38 approximated between ½ inch and 2 inches, whilst giving the opinion that they were not approximating.

The second group of subjects to be examined was a group of 49 schoolboy cadets, pre-OCTU, who were all aged 17. These boys were all of good intelligence, and were all in medical category A1. Without treating these observations in such detail as the previous ones, the following table gives a consolidation of observations 3, 4 and 5.

Observation 3 O-C approximation	*Observation 4* No.	Feeling	Abs't	*Observation 5* O-C approximation $\frac{1}{2}''$ and under	$1-\frac{1}{2}''$	$2-1''$	Over $2''$
$\frac{1}{2}$ inch and under	4	Yes	1	3	0	0	0
$\frac{1}{2}$ inch and under	1	No	0	1	0	0	0
1 inch—$\frac{1}{2}$ inch	17	Yes	1	6	10	0	0
1 inch—$\frac{1}{2}$ inch	15	No	2	6	7	0	0
2 inches—1 inch	5	Yes	0	0	3	2	0
2 inches—1 inch	5	No	0	2	2	1	0
Over 2 inches	1	Yes	0	0	1	0	0
Over 2 inches	0	No	0	0	0	0	0

The observations on this group of 49 schoolboy cadets showed that:

1 Out of 49 schoolboy cadets, all except one showed a greater or less degree of O-C approximation when sitting down in their usual unthinking manner, and of these only three were aware of the approximation when their attention was first drawn to it.

2 Out of 48 schoolboy cadets (excluding the one who showed no approximation), only four were able to prevent approximation when they tried.

3 Out of 48 schoolboy cadets, 28 stated that they could feel approximation occurring after their attention had been drawn to it. Of these 28, only two could prevent approximation occurring when they tried: the remaining 26 considered that they were preventing approximation occurring when they were in actual fact approximating between $\frac{1}{2}$ inch and 2 inches.

4 Out of 48 schoolboy cadets, 20 said they could not feel approximation occurring when their attention was focused on it and when they were seen to be approximating. When asked consciously to prevent approximation, 18 approximated between $\frac{1}{2}$ inch and 2 inches, whilst giving the opinion that they were not approximating.

Discussion
The relatively crude approach of the above investigation does not do justice to Alexander's conception of misuse and defective kinaesthesia. By our present standards, accustomed as we are to seeing and accepting as normal a considerable degree of distortion of form, the

misuse which Alexander describes may seem a relatively slight thing, and the untrained observer may not, at first, grasp what is entailed by it (see plates 10 and 11). It was possible, however, to show that in the group of cadets and schoolboy cadets under examination, Alexander's contention is borne out—that "in the activity of sitting down, in nearly all cases there is an alteration in the position of the head which is thrown back", and that in the majority of cases, the kinaesthesia was so untrustworthy a guide that it led them "to do the very opposite of what they wished to do or thought they were doing".

My thanks are due to Brigadier T. J. Ponting, MC, and to Lt.-Colonel K. G. Menzies, OBE, MC, for permission to carry out the above investigation, and to Captain M. Murray, RAMC, for assisting with the observations.

2 AN INVESTIGATION INTO POSTURAL DEFORMITY

Theoretical Aspects

Most of us, I think, are thoroughly dissatisfied with the results of posture training, whether it be carried out by the physical educationists or as remedial work. The incidence of defects in so-called "normals" is tremendous. The White House Conference put it as high as 75 per cent of adolescents: my own figure, based on over 500 students and members of the armed services, male and female, is higher than this. Of those who do make some initial improvement during the usual posture training, very few seem to want to maintain it after supervision has been stopped. This is partly because the wrong things are taught, and partly because of a quite wrong conception of the actual training process—the accent usually being on *instructing* the patient, instead of on how he is to *learn* something new. It is one thing to be instructed: quite another to change habits and learn.

Postural Homeostasis

In view of the undoubtedly unsatisfactory results of postural re-education, I suggested a few years ago that we should try to get rid of the usual idea of posture as being some fixed static position, which could either be good or bad, right or wrong; and, if bad and wrong, then caused by weakness of certain muscles, which needed strengthening through admonition, static holdings, and stretching and strengthening exercises. Instead I suggested the term "postural homeostasis", in order to give the idea of change and lack of fixity. I should like to elaborate this idea of postural homeostasis, on which my approach to postural re-education is based.

A homeostatic system is one which returns to a resting state of equilibrium when it is disturbed. Postural adjustment is a homeostatic mechanism which is largely under voluntary control, provided that the right amount of information about errors finds its way back from the muscle to the cortex.

Cannon's (1932) conception of homeostasis has become well known since he first put it forward 22 years ago. For an animal to remain alive, certain variables must remain within physiological limits. Body temperature, the blood glucose level, the blood pressure in the aorta, the volume of the circulating blood, are all examples of essential variables which must be maintained within narrow limits during adaptation to stress. The length of the nails or the length of the hair are other examples of variables which are not so essential to survival (except perhaps in the fashionable world of *haute couture*).

Cannon founded his theory of homeostasis on the type of circuit which involves "negative feed-back", the circuits on which Ashby (1952) and Wiener (1948) subsequently developed what is known as "Cybernetics". All negative feed-back circuits have this in common, that "they establish some particular state of the system, and they bring it back towards that state by an amount which increases with their deviation from that state". They are as we say "error-operated" (McCulloch, 1951). The employment of the feed-back principle means, in its simplest form, that "behaviour is scanned for its results, and the success or failure of this result modifies future behaviour" Weiner, 1950).

The typical feed-back circuit as applied to the central nervous system is shown simply in Fig. 4, which is adapted from Mackay (1951).

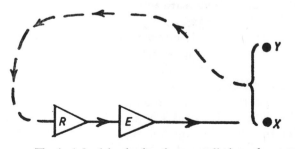

Figure 4. Typical feed-back circuit as applied to the central
nervous system

Here we are concerned with a goal-seeking movement or communication, in which X is the subject's current state, and Y is the state of subject+ environment which we call the goal. There must be an effector, E, capable of altering the state X, and this must be controlled by a receptor element, R, which is capable of receiving information and computing it against its previously stored experience. Information about the magnitude of XY must be fed back from the field of activity to R, thence to give rise after coding to activity in E leading to modification of the movement XY.

Steady Motion

Numbers of mechanical devices use this procedure—for example, the scanning mechanism required in television and radar, which scans an object as one might scan a printed page in search of a word. The thermostat is another example: when it corrects an error, it makes a new one, and this too it corrects by making a further but smaller error. It is in fact in a state of "steady motion": as the self-correcting mechanism over-shoots the mark, oscillation occurs. A similar stability based on a state of steady motion is shown by a top spinning on a vertical axis or a juggler balancing a number of objects on top of a pole. Riding a bicycle is another example (Wisdom, 1951). When the rider falls slightly to the right, he turns his front wheel to the right, which stops his fall but leads to his being thrown over on the left. This he corrects by turning his wheel to the left.

The state of stability which is achieved is the outcome of a multitude of compensating adjustments, and Cannon used his term homeostasis to include not only the state of steady motion but the processes leading to the state of steady motion. "In an open system such as our bodies represent, compounded of unstable material and subjected continuously to disturbing conditions, constancy is in itself evidence that agencies are acting or ready to act to maintain this constancy" (Cannon, 1932).

I use the term "postural homeostasis" to denote the state of steady motion which underlies all voluntary activity. Walshe (1951) has recently pointed out that oscillation is characteristic of all voluntary activity. Postural homeostasis in the intact organism is effected by feed-back from the eyes, the muscles, and the labyrinth, and the information which is fed back is assessed against the postural model —R in the diagram. During movement, disequilibrium signals are generated in the receptor R by incoming stimuli, causing activity through the effector E until there is a sufficient degree of resemblance between the incoming pattern and the postural model.

The Muscle Spindle System

It has been realized for many years that our main source of information about the amount of muscle tension we are exerting is the muscle spindle. Sherrington (1906) pointed out that the muscle spindle is, next to the eye and the ear, the third most elaborate sensory end-organ in the body; and we are all familiar with his classic description of the part played by the spindle in maintaining tonus, based on the stretch reflex which he described with Professor Liddell (Liddell and Sherrington, 1925). Sherrington did not, however, consider that he had given a clear account of postural tonus; in his own words: "The tonus of skeletal muscle is an obscure problem. Its mode of production, its distribution in the musculature, its purposive significance, are all debatable." In fact the classic Sherrington account has altered considerably, and Liddell (1954) drew attention to new work on the muscle spindle which appears to me to be of the greatest importance for those concerned with posture.

It has been known from as far back as 1842 that the motor roots of spinal nerves contain not only large nerve fibres with diameters, in man, of about 14 to 20 μ, but also a large group of much smaller nerve fibres, ranging from 10 μ to less than 3 μ in diameter, and making up between 25 per cent and 40 per cent of the total motor outflow. Recent practice is to call these two groups "large nerve fibres" and "small nerve fibres". Hunt and Kuffler (1951), following on the work of Matthews, have shown that the small nerve fibres are exclusively concerned with the innervation of the intrafusal muscles of the muscle spindle. Small nerve fibres do not go to the main extrafusal muscle fibres, and when stimulated they do not produce a muscle contraction. What does happen when they are stimulated is that the sensory discharge from the muscle spindle is appreciably increased; in fact, stimulation of the small nerve fibres *primes* the sensitivity of the muscle-spindle end-organ. If, however, muscle contraction is allowed to take place in the main muscle fibres, sensory discharge from the muscle spindle disappears, even when the small nerve fibres are stimulated. When a muscle is shortened spindle activity ceases. Since our detection of error in muscle tension is dependent on information coming from the spindle, this mechanism of spindle innervation is obviously of first-rate importance.

It can scarcely be doubted that this servo- or feed-back mechanism plays an essential part in the relatively minute moment-to-moment adjustments of normal muscular effort: and since spindle activity ceases when a muscle shortens, postural awareness will be hampered

by any activity which involves muscle-shortening, particularly if there
is not a quick return to the resting state of homeostasis.

The Resting State

Every homeostatic system has a resting state—a state of relative
stillness and constancy—to which it returns after disturbance. If we
very crudely depict the neurological analysis of behaviour into

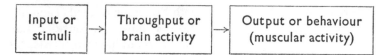

stability of reaction depends on both perception of "input" and
execution of "output" being carried out without too great a departure
from the resting state. It is the function of "throughput", or discriminate thinking, to maintain this resting state so that "errors" in
the input are noticed and so that output is released at the right time
and in the right serial order. We have all of us had the experience,
when waiting in a state of preparedness to carry out some activity, of
being set off ("tripped") by some inappropriate stimulus—some
accidental resemblance to the configuration which we are awaiting or
when we are very strung up, something which bears no resemblance
to it whatever. The ability to check a reaction to a stimulus and only
to release the response when we have decided the time is ripe requires
control over the "resting state". In anxiety states there is no such
control: there is a state of tense preparedness which is liable to
discharge excessively when the organism is stimulated; and in this
state, all manner of aspects of the environment are noticed and
reacted on, which would be ignored in a less tense state.

This resting state involves a co-ordinated distribution of muscle
tension throughout the various parts of the body. In practice it can
be shown that this co-ordinated distribution of tension depends
primarily on the correct management of the head-neck region, and it
is essential for such correct management (at the throughput level)
that the postural model should be accurate. (It is interesting that
Wittgenstein in his posthumously published book (1953) has a most
subtle analysis of problems of Will and Kinaesthesia, and quotes
William James as saying that "the self consists mainly of peculiar
motions in the head and between the head and throat".) The system
of postural modelling must enable us to notice and correct errors as
they occur: errors must be made as conspicuous as possible. Sir
Charles Bell, writing in 1852, enquired, "What then gives nobleness

and grace to the human form, and how is deformity to be avoided?'', and he came to the conclusion that a major factor was, "a deceptious sensibility as to the muscles". The problem of re-education is to replace this "deceptious sensibility" by something more reliable in the way of a postural modelling process.

The typical Pavlov conditioned reflex is well known, as are its deficiencies in explaining human behaviour. (Systems with feed-back cannot adequately be treated as if they were of one-way action, as Ashby points out.) Konorski (1949), the most prominent worker in this field at present, has described a second type of conditioned reflex, the "Konorski Type 2 reflex", as it is known. His description of it is: "If we subject to a conditioning procedure of the first type (the classical Pavlov type) a compound of stimuli consisting of an exteroceptive and proprioceptive stimulus, in which the proprioceptive stimulus constitutes an indispensable complement to the conditioned compound, then the exteroceptive stimulus begins to evoke the movement generating the proprioceptive stimulus." This sounds a little involved, but what it amounts to is that if you associate a given degree of muscle tension (and its associated feeling) with an external stimulus, in time this given tensional balance is produced by the external stimulus alone. Thorpe (1948) considers it a misnomer to call these reflexes conditioned reflexes, since "they represent a separate kind of plasticity. The response is an independent voluntary somatic action." Nevertheless, whether one terms them conditioned reflexes or not, this type of plasticity is shown by the nervous system, and can be employed as a basis of re-education.

The Alexander Technique

In carrying out re-education, I teach the subject to associate a verbal stimulus with an improved disposition of the body and its tensional balance. A sequence of such verbal orders is taught to the subject, and these orders are linked up for him by the teacher with the improved disposition of the body. The verbal orders are at first vocalized and then given subvocally as directions by the subject himself. The sequence of directions is designed to scan the body in serial order, and thus provides a postural model with both spatial and temporal co-ordinates. The important part in re-education, however, is to teach the subject not only *how* but *when* to release these guiding orders. For this reason it is essential to create a stimulus situation in which some action or communication is suggested as a goal and the subject is only permitted to respond to this situation when he has first canalized the response into the new behavioural sequence represented by the serial orders which he learns to give to himself. In this way he is enabled to detect errors in postural homeostasis which arise as he reacts on his environment, and to substitute at will a more balanced reaction.

This type of procedure was as far as I know first described by Alexander (1923). The above brief explanation of the procedure may seem a little complicated, but in practice it is readily understood by most people. Before describing the effect of its use on students, let us first enquire into the incidence of postural deformity.

Postural Deformity

Perhaps the best way to indicate the prevalence of postural deformity will be to give the results of a survey which I carried out at Dartford College, a college where a high physical standard is required at entry, and which draws on some of the best athletes and games players in the country. It can be reasonably claimed that this group of students have applied themselves from an early age to the development of their bodies, particularly in the gymnasium: and they are destined to become Physical Education teachers all over the country.

The entire group of first and second year students were photographed, using a squared background and a turntable which revolves into three standard positions. This ensures identical conditions, and the major postural faults show up as clearly as is possible under static conditions.

The faults can be analysed using Table I, and rated with 1, 2, or 3 "plusses" according to the severity of the fault. Many of the faults

TABLE I.—PROFORMA USED FOR SCORING POSTURAL FAULTS

Head	Poked, Retracted, Tilted, Pulled down
Shoulders	Raised, Dropped, Rotation, Pulled together
Pelvis	Tilt, Rotation, Forward carriage, Gluteal asymmetry
Spine	Scoliosis, Kyphosis, Lateral curvature or thorax displacement, Lordosis
Stance	Hyperextended knees, Int. rotation knees, Forward inclination, Symmetry
Tension	Specific, General

are reduplicated in the Table—a dropped shoulder is frequently the result of a lateral curvature which also may involve a head twist and a rotation of the pelvis, although each may occur separately. As far as is possible, a fault is only scored once. A given observer soon achieves a uniform pattern of scoring. My average scoring for the first and second year group only varied by 1 per cent which indicates that the method is accurate.

Analysing faults in this way, one soon finds a definite pattern appearing, of 5 well-defined categories—those scoring 0–3 faults who have excellent posture, those scoring 4–5 who have some slight defect, those between 6 and 9 faults who show moderately severe defects, those between 10 and 14 who show severe defects, and those over 15 who show really gross postural deformities. Fig. 5A shows an analysis of the 112 Physical Education students, and it will be seen that the majority—62 per cent—show a moderately severe defect, 11·5 per cent show a slight defect, and 26·5 per cent show a serious

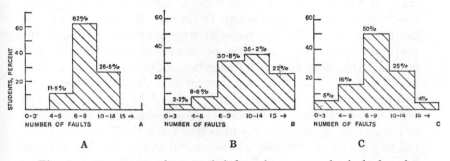

Figure 5. Percentage of postural defects in: A, 112 physical education students (females). B, 45 C.S.S. male students. C, 81 female drama students. 0–3 nil; 4–5 slight; 6–9 moderate; 10–14 severe; 15→ very severe

defect. There were no students in the top grade, and none in the lowest grade.

The students from the Physical Training College (Fig. 5A), show a high degree of mesomorphy (muscularity) in their Sheldon physique typing. If we turn to a group of male drama students, in whom the slender physique predominates, we find (Fig. 5B) an average of 11·2 faults: the curve has shifted appreciably to the right. An analysis of 81 female drama students (Fig. 5C) resembles the P.E. group more closely with an average of 8·0 faults, except that there are a few outstandingly good students and a few outstandingly bad ones. Since our purpose is to evaluate methods of educating posture, it is reasonable to begin by establishing the point that whatever methods are being used in our schools, the end-result even in the best students is not good.

Methods of Postural Re-education

The idea that a healthy natural outdoor life, with plenty of good food

D

and exercise, will ensure a reasonably good posture is not always true in my own experience, and we have seen how high is the incidence of defects in P.E. students. However, even if it were true, our main problem would still be how to establish a posture which will stand up to the strain of living in a civilization in which the healthy life may not be easily available.

There is much evidence to indicate that the methods of postural education and re-education employed in the past have not proved successful, and this in my view has been due to an over-simplification of the problem. The crux of the problem of postural control is the subject's *postural awareness*, and, at a different level, the *postural model* or *body schema* which the subject uses as a standard against which to detect his postural errors. In the past, too much reliance has been placed on verbal or pictorial instruction to re-educate the postural model, whilst the actual postural ability and its associated awareness has been tackled by exercises. Optimistically it has been hoped that people can "do what they are told", and that a little more will-power and "trying" is all that is required. Words and ideas will only become effective when they are accompanied by demonstration of the sensory experiences to which they refer. Such experience will not be given by an "exercise", as at present understood, but will only be learned after a period of conditioning in which the new model (verbal or otherwise) is associated with the appropriate degree of muscle tension, not only at rest but in preparation for movement, during movement, and after movement. In this way the subject learns a basic resting state of postural equilibrium which he can employ at will.

Comparison of Methods of Re-education
Some years ago a survey was carried out at the Central School of Speech in order to assess the efficacy of their methods of postural re-education. As a control group, I submitted a similar group of students from The Royal College of Music to the Alexander procedure in which a new postural model is linked to the correct experience of postural awareness. The Central School is a training college for speech therapists, speech teachers, and drama students, and is a good group to study since posture is considered by this school to be of fundamental importance throughout the whole three years' training. The principal had been dissatisfied with their results for some time, and she agreed that it was important for us to find out whether in fact their methods were being effective. One could sum up the methods employed at this school as being based on the giving of verbal instruction and occasional manual adjustment so that

the pupil would attempt to do the right thing to correct the posture when a teacher noticed it was wrong. Thus if a shoulder was dropped, the student would be told to correct it by holding it up, and might receive exercises to strengthen the dropped side: if the head was pulled back, the student was told to put it forward, and so on. No attempt was made at a conditioning procedure, and it was taken for granted that if a fault was pointed out and perhaps manually corrected, the student would then be able to maintain the correction. To promote general awareness of posture and movement, great use was made of a form of exercise introduced by Laban, known as "The Art of Movement", a method much advocated at the recent Ling Conference on School Gymnastics.

In spite of this constant preoccupation with posture at the Central School, the average number of faults in 25 girls at the start of training was 7·5: at the end of training it was 7·9. The average number of faults in 19 men at the start was 10·6: at the end 11·7. In fact deterioration had taken place.

For comparison, the group of students from The Royal College of Music were trained by the Alexander procedure. In this group, the average number of faults in thirteen men before re-education was eleven; at the end five. In seventeen girls, the average number of faults was nine before training; at the end it was four. This represents a considerable improvement. A detailed comparison of the Central School and Royal College students is shown in Fig. 6A (female) and Fig. 6B (male).

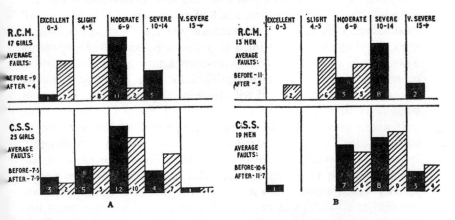

Figure 6. Comparison of re-educational methods. Improvement in RCM students, deterioration in CSS students (A) female, (B) male. Black blocks = numbers before. Striped blocks = numbers after training.

This experiment makes it clear that postural re-education will be ineffective unless a new "body schema" is taught, by associating the postural model with an improved postural awareness.

Physiotherapeutic Methods

Turning to a consideration of methods at present used by many Physical Medicine Departments, perhaps the commonest method used by physiotherapists is a combination of exercise and "static holding". "In treating the patient with a postural defect, static holdings are carefully taught and the patient encouraged to feel the sense of the good posture. It is form of muscle contraction which is said to re-educate the postural reflex. By repeated and concentrated holdings, an appreciation of the new posture is established."

This quotation from a physiotherapy textbook is a typical example of current methods. Such methods must be considered from the point of view of whether they increase postural awareness. I have suggested previously that the muscle spindle mechanism, which mediates much of our postural sense, is put out of action by excessive muscular contraction. It is always hazardous to transfer the results of animal physiology to the human, but there seems to be fairly clear agreement now that postural feed-back from the muscle is more effective when a muscle lengthens than when it shortens; it is difficult to see how the "holding" and over-contraction of muscle can help to promote postural awareness. Moreover, the connection between excessive muscular contraction and states of anxiety, in which the excessive contraction produces a lack of awareness of the body, is well established. I think it can be reasonably stated that the teaching of muscular contraction as a form of postural re-education to patients who already exhibit muscular over-contraction and an inability to return to a resting state of equilibrium after activity, will only accentuate the problem and will decrease the patient's awareness of what he is doing.

It might be said that these contraction exercises "strengthen the back muscles", but this is based on a faulty conception of "strength". Inman (1952) has shown that the *longer* the resting length of a muscle, the greater the force exerted and the less the electromyographic activity which accompanies it. The "strength" to maintain adequate postural relationships at rest and during movement does not come from muscle-shortening and over-contraction, but from maintaining a correct equilibrium between the various parts of the body. To attain this equilibrium, the patient needs to be taught to release superfluous muscular tension and return to a resting state in which the muscles are lengthening.

I should like to define the word "posture" as "A person's willingness and ability to maintain that relationship of the different parts of his body which ensures their most efficient behavioural function and physiological functioning both now and in the future." Such a definition underlines the fact that posture is a psychosomatic affair, in which habit plays a part, and that "good posture" does not imply some ideal standard, but rather a person's willingness and ability to maintain the best relationship possible for *him*, whether or not there may be some pathology present. The psychosomatic basis of postural deformity becomes apparent to anyone who works for long in this field, for as we proceed with our training, we encounter definite psychological obstacles—habits, attitudes and dispositions to which the patient is profoundly attached and which he is reluctant to change. I have mentioned these problems before (1955*a*). One soon finds that postural awareness occupies a key position in determining a person's idea of himself, and that as this awareness alters, profound alterations may take place in habits of thought.

It will be seen that the aim of re-education is to teach the patient a basic "resting state" which he can achieve even when under stress. Other methods which are used to achieve relaxation, seem to me to fall short. My experience of these methods is that someone certainly may be taught to relax under ideal conditions: but as soon as he becomes active again, the old tension pattern returns. He has not been taught to check his overquick input-output response and to employ discriminate thinking (throughput) and he has not been given an operational standard which will inform him as soon as he begins to make tension again. He has, in fact, been treated as a "one-way" system, ignoring the presence of feed-back. It is not until he has acquired a sense of the amount of unconscious "pressure" which he exerts in moving himself and in handling his environment that he will be able to maintain a requisite balance of tension. And it is not until he learns to notice the extent to which he interferes with his postural homeostasis during performance that he will have a chance of achieving what Henry James called "The perfect presence of mind, unconfused, unhurried by emotion."

APPLICATIONS

PSYCHOLOGICAL

NINE

Preoccupation with the Disconnected
by John Dewey

THE VERY PROBLEM of mind and body suggests division; I do not know of anything so disastrously affected by the habit of division as this particular theme. In its discussion are reflected the splitting off from each other of religion, morals and science; the divorce of philosophy from science and of both from the arts of conduct. The evils which we suffer in education, in religion, in the materialism of business and the aloofness of "intellectuals" from life, in the whole separation of knowledge and practice—all testify to the necessity of seeing mind-body as an integral whole.

The division in question is so deep-seated that it has affected even our language. We have no word by which to name mind-body in a unified wholeness of operation. For if we said "human-life" few would recognize that it is precisely the unity of mind and body in action to which we were referring. Consequently, when we endeavour to establish this unity in human conduct, we still speak of body *and* mind and thus unconsciously perpetuate the very division we are striving to deny.

I have used, in passing, the phrases "wholeness of operation", "unity in action". What is implied in them gives the key to the discussion. In just the degree in which *action, behaviour*, is made central, the traditional barriers between mind and body break down and dissolve. When we take the stand-point of action we may still treat some functions as primarily physical and others as primarily mental. Thus we think of, say, digestion, reproduction and locomotion as conspicuously physical, while thinking, desiring, hoping, loving, fearing are distinctively mental. Yet if we are wise we shall not regard the difference as other than one of degree and emphasis.

If we go beyond this and draw a sharp line between them, consigning one set to body exclusively and the other to mind exclusively, we are at once confronted by undeniable facts. The being who eats and digests is also the one who at the same time is sorrowing and rejoicing; it is a commonplace that he eats and digests in one way to one effect when glad, and in another when he is sad. Eating is also a social act, and the emotional temper of the festal board enters into the alleged merely physical function of digestion. Eating of bread and drinking of wine have indeed become so integrated with the mental attitudes of multitudes of persons that they have assumed a sacramental spiritual aspect.

There is no need to pursue this line of thought to other functions which are sometimes termed exclusively physical. The trouble is that instead of taking the act in its entirety we cite the multitude of relevant facts only as evidence of influence of mind on body and of body on mind, thus starting from and perpetuating the idea of their independence and separation even when dealing with their connection. What the facts testify to is not an influence exercised across and between two separate things, but to behaviour so integrated that it is artificial to split up into two things.

The more human and civilized mankind becomes, the less is there some behaviour which is purely physical and some other which is purely mental. So true is this statement that we may use the amount of distance which separates them in our society as a test of the degree of human development in a given community. There exists in present society, especially in industry, a large amount of activity that is almost exclusively mechanical; that is, carried on with a minimum of thought and of accompanying emotion. There is a large amount of activity, especially in "intellectual" and "religious" groups, in which the physical factor is at a minimum and what little there is is regretted as a deplorable necessity. But either sort of behaviour in the degree of its onesidedness marks a degradation, an acquired habit whose formation is due to undesirable conditions; each marks an approximation to the pathological, a departure from that wholeness which is health. When behaviour is reduced to a purely physical level and a person becomes like a part of the machine he operates, there is proof of social maladjustment. This is reflected in the disordered and defective habits of the persons who act on the merely physical plane.

Action does not cease to be abnormal because it is said to be spiritual and concerned with ideal matters—too refined to be infected with gross matter. Nor is it enough that we should recognize the part played by brain and nervous system in making our highly intellectual and "spiritual" activities possible. It is equally important that we realize that the latter are truncated and tend towards abnormality in the degree that they do not eventuate in employing and directing physical instrumentalities to effect material changes. Otherwise, that which is called spiritual is in effect but indulgence in idle fantasy.

Thus the question of integration of mind-body in action is the most practical of all questions we can ask of our civilization. It is not just a speculative question, it is a demand—a demand that the labour of multitudes now too predominantly physical in character be inspired by purpose and emotion and informed by knowledge and understanding. It is a demand that what now pass for highly intellectual functions shall be integrated with the ultimate conditions and means of all achievement, namely the physical, and thereby accomplish something beyond themselves. Until this integration is effected in the only place where it can be carried out, in action itself, we shall continue to live in a society in which a soulless and heartless materialism is compensated for by soulful but futile idealism and spiritualism.

We need to distinguish between action that is routine and action that is alive with purpose and desire; between that which is cold, and that which is warm and sympathetic; between that which marks a withdrawal from the conditions of the present and that which faces actualities; between that which is expansive and developing (because including what is new and varying) and that which applies only to the uniform and repetitious; between that which is bestial and that which is godlike in its humanity; between that which is spasmodic and centrifugal, dispersive and dissipating, and that which is centred and consecutive.

Until we can make such distinctions, and make them in a multitude of ways and degrees, we shall not be able to understand the conduct of individuals, and not understanding, shall not be able to help them in the management of their lives. Because of this lack, education will be a guess in the dark, business a gamble in shifting-about and circulating material commodities, and politics an intrigue in manipulation. What most stands in the way of our achieving a working technique for making such discriminations and employing them in the guidance of the actions of those who stand in need of assistance is our habit of splitting up the qualities of action into two disjoined things.

F. M. Alexander has pointed out that until we have a procedure in actual practice which demonstrates the continuity of mind and body, we shall increase the disease in the means used to cure it. Those who talk most of the organism, physiologists and psychologists, are often just those who display least sense of the intimate, delicate and subtle interdependence of all organic structures and processes with one another. The world seems mad in pre-occupation with what is specific, particular and disconnected in medicine, politics, science, industry and education.

We are reminded of happier days when the divorce of knowledge and action, theory and practice, had not been decreed, and when the arts, as action informed by knowledge, were not looked down upon in invidious disparagement with contemplation complete in itself; when knowledge and reason were not so "pure" that they were defiled by entering into the wider connections of an action that accomplishes something because it uses physical means. In Greece, there was a time when philosophy, science and the arts, medicine included, were much closer together than they have been since. One word described both science and art—*techné*.

There are signs that we are perforce, because of the extension of knowledge on one side and the demands of practice on the other, about to attempt a similar achievement on our own account. The growing interest in pre-school education, nursery schools and parental education, the development of medical inspection, the impact of social hygiene, and the use of schools as social centres are all evidence that the isolation of schools from life is beginning to give way. But not even the most optimistic would hold that we have advanced beyond the outer breastworks. The forces are still powerful that make for divisive education. And the chief of these is, let it be repeated, the separation of mind and body which is incarnated in religion, morals and business as well as in science and philosophy. The full realization of the integration of mind and body in action waits upon the reunion of philosophy and science in the supreme art of education.

TEN

Anxiety and Muscle Tension
by Dr Wilfred Barlow

ALEXANDER'S WORK on muscle tension and its re-education became part of an upsurge of interest in psychophysical correlates during the years between world war I and world war II. The following paper is an amalgam of two papers which I wrote soon after world war II, both of them with the title, "Anxiety and Muscle Tension", and both of them intended to bring the Alexander Technique into line with other anatomical and physiological work at that time.

The Anxiety State

"Anxiety state" became a familiar label during world war II. The psychiatrists describe it as differing from "fear" in that "fear" is a reasonable reaction to a harmful situation. "Anxiety state", however, is a state of worrying about "you don't know what". You wake up in the morning in a worrying state, and you hasten through the day's work leaving a trail of havoc behind you. Periods of frantic "doing", alternate with even longer periods of complete prostration. Temporary relief appears to come from "getting things done", only to be followed by periods of headache, irritation and despair. Periods of rest may give some relief, but the trouble usually recurs when an active life is resumed.

Anxiety has been termed the *mal du siècle*, and most of us are familiar with it both in its objective and subjective forms. The condition is, in fact, so familiar to the man in the street that it has tended in recent years to be written up not so much by the medical fraternity as by the general writer. The words *"Angst"* and *"Angoisse"* (anxiety) are familiar coinage amongst, for example, the existentialists, and Cyril Connolly was writing in 1945:

> I wake up in anxiety: like a fog it overlaps all I do, and my days are muffled in anguish. I dread the bell, the post, the telephone, the sight of an aquaintance. . . . We know very little about *Angst*, which may even proceed from the birth trauma, or be a primitive version of original sin. Freudians consider anxiety to arise from

the repression of anger or love, Theologians associate it with the Fall, Behaviourists with undigested food in the stomach, Kierkegaard with the vertigo that precedes sin. Buddha and many philosophers regarded it as concurrent with desire. *Angst* is inherent in the uncoiling of the ego: it lurks in old loves, in old letters and in our despair at the complexity of modern life.

It is not surprising that in recent years we have seen a flood of what Mr Connolly called "blue-sky books"—books of a general nature which aim at counteracting some of the stress and anxiety of modern life. A few years ago, the four top-selling new books in the United States of America fell into this category, and we do not have to look far into the advertisement columns of our own national press to find such titles as *Stop that Worrying Tension, Relax Yourself Inside, Get Right with Your Spine*, and so on. (These titles are all fictitious as far as I know.) A thorough survey of this field would, in fact, have to take in a vast range of activities which hover on the periphery of medicine. *Westernized Yoga* (Coster, 1934), chiropraxis, and such curiosities as *Semantic Relaxation* (Johnson, 1946) can all be said to be to some extent concerned with what I call "moral physiology"—the pre-occupation of mind with muscle—and they muster a considerable following among intelligent members of society.

Rest, Relaxation and Re-education

The ancient world recognized that bodily care was a basic social responsibility, and the earliest ideas of relaxation of tension seem usually to have been connected with the bath. The Mycenean bath in which the homeric heroes bathed was looked on as a restorative after "soul-exhausting toil". The Roman work day, which began at dawn and ended at midday, often included a visit after work to the *thermae* for a combination of exercise and hydrotherapeutic relaxation. The Greek gymnasium had a similar function, although repose and relaxation came increasingly to be separated, in the *exedra*, from the more vigorous activities of the *palestra*. This separation of relaxation from exercise was even more accentuated in the *hammam*, or Islamic bath, where there was "half light, quiescence, and seclusion from the outside world" (Gideon, 1948). Varying ages have accentuated either the active or the passive side of personal recreation, and there persists in our time a conflict between those who believe in offsetting the wear and tear of civilization by hardening the body, and those who seek repose in the heat of a Turkish bath or the theatre.

In discussing rest and relaxation it is customary to mention the pioneer work of Weir Mitchell (1908), who drew attention to the fact that neurotic patients could be benefited by a definite régime of rest and physical therapy, including a light stroking massage given over the entire body to induce relaxation. It should also be remembered that the continuous tepid bath has been used extensively in psychiatric institutions as a means of producing muscular relaxation in maniacal patients. I do not, however, propose to discuss here such methods, nor the use of muscle-relaxing drugs, but to mention briefly work which involves a training of the patient, and which, for lack of a better title, is usually referred to as re-education.

There are a number of such methods which have as their basic principle what Kretschmer (1951) described as "the induced regulation of tonus". In giving his approval to such methods, he claimed that, "the majority of neuroses, even complicated cases, respond to this kind of treatment, with a great saving of time and energy". In the past Jacobson's (1938) "progressive relaxation" has been used widely by physiotherapists, and Krusen (1951) gives a good shortened account of it. Recently the application of Jacobson's work to the neuroses has been admirably outlined by Garmany (1953). Garmany's work is addressed primarily to physiotherapists, and gives an excellent outline of the relationship between emotional disturbances and muscle tension. One should also perhaps mention here the work of Reich (1949) on the dissolution of muscle-armouring, and the writings of Fink (1945) and Rathbone (1936). Various psychoanalysts from Groddeck onward have used massage and relaxation to help promote rapport with the patient, and the connection between relaxation and hypnotic phenomena has been described by Salter (1950), who has a method of auto-hypnosis approved by Dr E. B. Strauss. On the continent of Europe perhaps the best known method is that of Schultz (1952), consisting in relaxation and "directed attention" exercises aimed at giving control over the automatic nervous system. In his address at the Royal Society of Medicine, this was the method which Kretschmer (1951) described himself as using, and he concluded: "These training methods have a special practical application in the field of psychosomatic medicine ... applicable to all disorders which depend directly or indirectly on a disequilibrium of the automatic centres and their endocrine connections."

Without wishing to deny the benefits to be derived from these various re-educational approaches, they seem to me to fall short for a number of reasons, which I will discuss below.

The Distribution of Muscle Tension

Many of these re-educational techniques have originated in departments of physiotherapy, along with more active methods of teaching muscle control. I have no wish to revive here the vitalist-mechanist controversy but it is interesting to note that physiotherapy in Great Britain still takes an almost outright mechanist view. Lorenz (1950) summed it up delightfully by saying that, when a dog walks, the mechanist thinks it is the leg which moves the dog, whilst the vitalist thinks it is the dog which moves the leg. Physiotherapy mostly takes the view that it is "the leg which moves the dog", and re-education proceeds on the basis of training specific muscles without reference to the effect of such training on the whole organism.

Marcus Aurelius asked himself 1,800 years ago, "What then is valuable?", and concluded that the goal of all training was "movement, and abstention from movement". Physiotherapy has seen no reason to disagree with the literal interpretation of this, and it is within the overall framework of "movement" that physiotherapy carries out its training activities. It is, however, apparent that the human organism, in its muscular activity, is not merely concerned with cleaving a pathway through space. In addition to moving itself, the organism moves and manipulates its environment; most important of all when we are considering anxiety states, the organism communicates with other organisms.

In considering muscle tension, we have in fact to deal not only with movement but with behaviour, and when we come to re-educate the patient, it is necessary to consider the question of the distribution of muscle tension throughout the whole body during behaviour and during thought.

The Anxiety State and Muscle Tension

For many years I have been struck by this intimate relationship between states of anxiety and observable states of muscular tension— *"pas de pensée sans expression"*, or, in Ribot's phrase, *"tout état intellectuel est accompagné de manifestations physiques determinées"*. It is not a particularly novel idea, but it is one which has been brought to the fore by the recent accent on "psychosomatic medicine". In a review in the *British Medical Journal* of Flanders Dunbar's book on that subject (Dunbar, 1945), it was said: ". . . the degree and type of the patient's muscular tension . . . may be revealing if sometimes difficult to evaluate. Such tensions . . . can express themselves in visceral as well as in somatic muscles, thus producing organic symptoms."

If one suggests that, on the one hand, tension may produce symptoms of autonomic imbalance and that, on the other hand, anxiety may produce similar symptoms, then one has to consider whether a therapeutic approach directed towards the inculcation of an ability to control consciously the muscular tension may not get right to the heart of the problem of the psychosomatic disease. I am using loosely the phrase "an ability to control consciously the muscular tension", and an attempt to elaborate it is made below.

When I first stressed this connection (1947) psychiatric opinion as typified by Gregg (1944) was that, in anxiety "no structural or chemical variation is known to accompany in characteristic fashion the all too obvious symptoms": and in discussing "the long list of psychoneurotics with their hysterias, anxieties, obsessions and states of inexplicable fatigue and indecision", he concluded that, "in none of these conditions is there any characteristic physical accompaniment which can be detected by present methods".

Since that time, electromyographic techniques have made it clear (Wolff, 1948; Sainsbury and Gibson, 1954; Malmo and others, 1949; Barlow, 1954) that muscular over-activity occurs in patients complaining of anxiety and tension. Sainsbury, using an electronic integrator to pick up muscle potentials via surface electrodes, showed such a method to be statistically consistent, and Malmo found a correlation between, for example, unconscious hostility and arm tension, and between leg tension and sexual themes. One may quote Sainsbury's finding that patients with what was once considered to be a typical neurotic complaint of a feeling of tension over the scalp, can in fact be shown electromyographically to be tensing the scalp musculature: and perhaps the most striking observation has been that of Wolff, who in his exhaustive textbook on *Headache*, found that by far the largest group of any patients was made up of those with "marked contraction of muscles in the neck. Such sustained contraction may be secondary to noxious impulses arising from disease of any structure in the head: more common, however, are the sustained contractions associated with emotional strain, dissatisfaction, apprehension and anxiety."

The point of view which I am putting forward here, is that when a man is worrying, he is carrying out his worrying activity through the manner in which he uses his muscular mechanisms, and that we can observe, in the manner in which he uses his muscular mechanisms, "a structural variation which accompanies in characteristic fashion the all too obvious symptoms". I am suggesting that worrying is associated with neuromuscular activity, and that the habitually recurrent pattern of worry which characterizes the psychoneurotic has its basis in a habitual pattern of muscular tensions.

I do not claim any great originality in putting forward this suggestion; many years ago William James (1915) was writing at length on the subject: "By the sensations that so incessantly pour from the over-tensed, excited body, the over-tense and excited habit of mind is kept up; and the sultry, threatening, exhausting, thunderous inner atmosphere never quite clears away."

My own ideas on the subject are derived from the teaching of F. M. Alexander, who developed the logical next step from this thesis. Following his teaching, I am suggesting that the habit of worrying can be detected in the manner of use of the muscular mechanisms—it may be a delicate and subtle level of activity—and that it may therefore be dealt with by an approach which seeks to raise to the level of consciousness the habitual underlying pattern of muscular tension (Alexander 1932). Before I indicate the way in which Alexander developed this thesis, however, I should like to make a digression in order to consider other approaches which have been made in the past to a study of "the pattern of muscular tension".

Studies in Muscular Tension
An account of previous work on this subject is extremely difficult to present in a coherent framework, but for present purposes I am dividing it up into (1) relatively *gross* studies of muscle action which have been carried out by physical anthropologists, anatomists and orthopaedists, and (2) relatively *fine* studies of muscle action which have been carried out by neurophysiologists and neuropsychiatrists.

Anthropological Studies
The physical anthropologists have always been concerned with posture. As Professor Wood Jones (1910) said:

> Different anatomists have assigned varying importance to the upright posture and its accompanying blessings. Among the earlier of them it was customary to see something very distinctive—typically human if not partially divine—in the posture, "that majestic attitude which announces his superiority over all the other inhabitants of the globe". That the upright habit is of the very first importance as an evolutionary factor must be freely admitted.

In the writings of Sir Arthur Keith, author of the classic study on man's posture, we get the view that the stress which civilized life imposes upon man's posture and muscular pattern of action is responsible for many serious ills:

It is not true to say that our spines are not perfectly adapted to the upright posture: it would be more accurate to say that human spines were not evolved to withstand the monotonous and trying positions entailed by modern education and by many modern industries. . . . We shall be wise to seek in these modern conditions of life for the factors which contribute to our liability to [hernia]. Two of these modern factors solicit the attention of medical men. The first of these is the states of high pressure which arise within the abdominal cavities of modern labourers during violent effort, as in lifting heavy weights, or in the physically weak during acts of coughing or straining at stool. On standing up, the pressure on the floor of the pelvis, taken from within the passive rectum, varies from about 15 to 25 mm. of mercury so long as we stand still, but the moment we attempt any arm movement, particularly if we bend down and seek to lift a heavy weight, the intra-pelvic pressure, as registered on a manometer, instantly rises to the neighbourhood of 80 to 100 mm. If the effort is made suddenly, the initial rise is much greater, reaching as much as 150 mm. In all such movements the visceral contents of the abdomen are compressed within the envelope of the postural musculature and seek out the weakest points in the containing walls. No one will deny that modern civilization has increased the abdominal strain for labouring men and women.

Likewise Dr Hooton, Professor of Anthropology at Harvard, and author of *Why Men behave like Apes, and vice versa*, wrote in 1936:

Man is a made-over animal. The bony framework has been warped and cramped and stretched in one part or another, in accordance with variations in the stresses and strains put upon it by different postures and changes in body bulk. Joints devised for mobility have been re-adapted for stability. Muscles have had violence done to their origins and insertions, and have suffered enormous inequalities in the distribution of labour. Viscera have been pushed hither and yon, hitched up, let down, reversed and inverted.

These brief quotations from the anthropologists may show that they have studied the pattern of muscle action from the anatomical point of view, chiefly in its effect upon the bony framework; they have studied on the one hand the part which it plays in posture, and on the other hand the effect which muscular distortion of the bony framework may have upon the underlying organs and tissues. There is a fairly common agreement among them that civilized life may set up new problems with which man's instinctive pattern of muscle action may not be able to cope.

Orthopaedic Studies

This anatomical approach has also been adopted by the orthopaedists. "The speciality known as Orthopaedics deals, in some degree, with bodily difficulties due to man's imperfect adaptation to an erect posture and to a biped mode of progression" (Hooton, 1936). Nevertheless, as practising surgeons, the orthopaedists have been been more concerned than have the anthropologists with what they should do about it for the benefit of their patients. Chief among the orthopaedists who studied the problem was Goldthwait, who, in his article in 1915, "An Anatomic and Mechanistic Conception of Disease", and later in his book, *Body Mechanics in Health and Disease* (1934), took as his thesis that, "an individual is in the best possible health only when the body is used so that there is no strain on any of its parts". The following quotation gives a brief review of his ideas.

When the body is used rightly, all of the structures are in such adjustment that there is no particular strain in any part. The physical processes are at their best, the mental functions are performed most easily, and the personality or spirit of the individual possesses its greatest strength. If the body is drooped or relaxed, so that the shoulders drag forward and downward, the whole body suffers, the weight is thrown imperfectly upon the feet so that the arch must be strained; the knees are slightly sprung, which shows by the crepitating joints; the pelvis is changed in its inclination, with strain to the sacroiliac joints and low back. The increased forward curve of the upper dorsal spine results not only in strain to the interspinous ligaments, but also forces the shoulders forward, with frequent irritation of the bursae about the shoulder, or compression of the brachial plexus, with pain and neuralgias in the arms, while the craning forward of the head must result in strain to the posterior part of the cervical spine. In this position the chest is necessarily lowered, the lungs are much less fully expanded than normal, the diaphragm is depressed, the abdominal wall is relaxed, so that with the lessened support of the abdominal wall together with the lowering of the diaphragm the abdominal organs are necessarily forced downward and forward. When this occurs, the possibility of mechanical interference with the functions of the organs is not difficult to imagine, and it becomes apparently a mere matter of chance which organ is affected. The thing which is important in the interpretation of the many symptoms which the patients describe is that the body is intimately related in all its different parts, so that no one part can be used wrongly without the body as a whole suffering. Once the foregoing conception of health and disease is grasped, the treatment for the individual case naturally consists first of all in correcting faulty mechanics so that the different structures may be able to work as near to normal as possible.

A Link between Orthopaedics and Neuropsychiatry

The orthopaedic approach has chiefly concerned itself with an anatomical diagnosis in terms of bone and joint mechanics. More recent writers on the subject, however, have found difficulty in eliminating psychological considerations from their approach. They have, in fact, been moving in the direction of the second broad group into which I divide the studies of "the pattern of muscle action" —the work which I group under that of neurophysiologists and neuropsychiatrists. To show this transition in the orthopaedic approach, let me quote from two papers by Sweet (1938) and by Le Vay (1947).

Sweet follows very much Goldthwait's account of the influence of poor body mechanics upon functioning, but is also concerned with the subject's awareness of the way in which he is using himself mechanically.

When faults in body mechanics become sufficiently great, the stress causes pain, but long before the threshold of pain is reached, the nervous system is irritated to a highly unfavourable degree. All deformities tend to increase: the deformity allows the shortening and gain in strength of muscles over their opponents: *any posture or method of movement tends to become implanted in the kinaesthetic sense as a habit*: generally it is easier and more comfortable to rest and move with a deformity than against it towards correction.

Le Vay (1947) has as his general purpose the following:

> . . . to show that psychological factors are often the cause of what
> is usually regarded as gross orthopaedic physical disease, and that
> emotions may greatly modify muscular tension, posture and even
> osseous structure. . . . Observation and introspection both confirm
> the intimate reflection of the emotional state of the mind on the
> tonus of skeletal and visceral muscle.

It will be seen that this is in accordance with my general thesis,
that anxiety and muscle tension are intimately bound up with each
other. Le Vay described in his article the work of Jacobson in the
United States of America. Jacobson developed a method of estimating
by means of skin electrodes the effects of *imagined* movements; when
an actual movement is carried out, the skin electrodes will pick up
the action currents passing to the muscle from its nerve; when the
movement is imagined but not actually carried out, Jacobson claims
to be able to find these self-same action currents recorded. "The
practical point emerging is the impossibility of conceiving an activity
without causing fine contractions in all those muscles which produce
that activity in reality." This is what Le Vay calls "the *kinaesthetic
equivalent*" of a movement—"the remembered experience of using
these muscles which is an indispensable preliminary to the movement
in reality". He goes on to suggest that postural tonus is the end
result of the individual's struggle with repressed emotion: ". . . hence
normal erect posture may be modified. Stooping and submissive
postures are derived from feelings of abasement and abandonment,
and other postures may resemble gestures of defence and defiance.
The whole body may be regarded as an organ of expression which
which can be deformed by the inner current of emotion." This was
well known to older psychologists, and William James's comment
was: "Thus the sovereign voluntary path to cheerfulness, if our
spontaneous cheerfulness be lost, is to sit up cheerfully, and to act
and speak as if cheerfulness were already there" (James, 1915).

It will be seen from the above that some, at least of the orthopaedists, have found difficulty in helping their patients without taking
into account psychological factors. They have found that "the kinaesthetic equivalent of movement"—the pattern of neuro-muscular
co-ordination which has been established in the past and which
constitutes the "know-how" of movement—cannot be disregarded
when they attempt to "correct faulty mechanics so that the different
structures may be able to work as near to normal as possible".

Neuropsychiatric Studies
Sir Charles Sherrington in 1946 described from the neurological point of view just why the orthopaedist, when he wishes to "correct faulty mechanics", runs into difficulties.

It is largely the reflex element in the willed movement of posture which, by reason of its unconscious character, defeats our attempts to know the "how" of the doing of even a willed act. Breathing, standing, walking, sitting, although innate, along with our growth, are apt, as movements, to suffer from defects in our ways of doing them. A chair unsuited to a child can quickly induce special and bad habits of sitting and breathing. In urbanized and industrialized communities, bad habits in our motor acts are especially common. But verbal instruction as to how to correct wrong habits of movement and posture is very difficult. The scantiness of our sensory perception of how we do them makes it so. The faults tend to escape our direct observation and recognition. Of the proprioceptive reflexes as such, whether of muscle or ear, we are unconscious. Subjective projection, instead of indicating, blinds the place of their objective source. Correcting the movements carried out by our proprioceptive reflexes is something like trying to reset a machine whose works are intangible. Instruction in such an act has to fall back on other factors more accessible to sense. To watch another performer trying the movement can be helpful; or a looking-glass in which to watch ourselves trying it. The mirror can often tell us more than the most painstaking attempt to introspect. Mr Alexander has done a service to the subject by insistingly treating each act as involving the whole integrated individual, the whole psycho-physical man. To take a step is an affair, not of this or that limb solely, but of the total neuro-muscular activity of the moment—not least of the head and neck.

With this quotation from Sir Charles Sherrington I close my digression in order to resume my account of the teaching of F. M. Alexander. This digression is only a sketch and scarcely touches on the vast amount of work which has been done, particularly in the neurological and psychological fields, but it may serve to set Alexander's work in perspective.

The Head-neck Relationship to the Body
Sherrington's closing words, "not least of the head and the neck",

can serve as a starting point. Alexander's writings will be found to
have much in common with the "body mechanics" school. There is
the same insistence on the close relationship which exists between
the manner of use of the muscular mechanisms and the standard of
functioning:

> . . . for where I have found unsatisfactory use of the mechanisms,
> the functional trouble associated with it has included interference
> with the respiratory and circulatory systems, dropping of the
> abdominal viscera, sluggishness of various organs, together with
> undue and perverted pressures, contractions and rigidities through-
> out the organism, all of which tend to lower the standard of
> resistance to disease (Alexander, 1932).

Unlike the "body mechanics" school, however, Alexander's
conception of what constitutes a satisfactory body mechanics puts an
especial accent on the neuro-muscular activity of the head and neck.
Alexander claims that unless the mechanical use of this region is
free and unimpeded, it is impossible to remedy defects in the rest
of the organism without fear of relapse. In accentuating this point,
he is only bringing to light what is already recognized in the
fields of anatomy and physiology, as the following quotations will
show.

> Goldthwait has pointed out that the viscera are slung from the
> cervical fascia by way of the attachment of the pericardium to the
> diaphragm and the diaphragmatic attachments of the abdominal
> viscera. Only when the dorsal and cervical portions of the spine are
> fully extended are the viscera raised to the best functional level.
> The position of greatest economy, which at the same time allows
> fullest play of the shoulder and arm muscles, is therefore the fully
> erect position with the neck line perpendicular (Sweet, 1938).

> The quadruped holds up his head by means of a powerful liga-
> mentum nuchae which is aided by strong posterior neck muscles.
> In the human being, however, the skull is delicately balanced on
> the cervical spine. The ligamentum nuchae is rudimentary and the
> neck muscles act like guy ropes. . . . The stomach is attached to the
> diaphragm at the cardia, and the pyloric end is fixed to the body
> wall. The liver is partially suspended from the diaphragm, and the
> transverse colon indirectly by means of the mesocolon. A great
> load is therefore carried by the centre of the diaphragm, which at

least partially is held through the right pericardium by the continuation of the cervical fascia (Hansson, 1945).

In the man of average weight, the shoulders and arms represent a burden of about 20 lbs. They are suspended from the cervical and upper dorsal regions of the spine, chiefly by the trapezius muscle. The essential circumstance which gives rise to plexus pressure is the failure or partial failure of the mechanism evolved for the support of the shoulders in the erect posture (Keith, 1923).

Whenever the cervical spine is strengthened the deep fascia of the neck is made tense, and through its attachment to the pericardium and thereby to the central tendon of the diaphragm, it acts as a suspensory ligament to that muscle and to the heart (Forrester-Brown, 1926).

Discussing the controlling influence exerted by the head-neck relationship upon the attitude of the rest of the body, Professor Magnus wrote in his Croonian and Cameronian lectures, in 1925 and 1926:

A very finely elaborated control apparatus is needed to combine and distribute all the afferent (incoming) impulses, depending on and adapted to the always changing circumstances of environment. Most important are the general attitudinal reflexes by which the whole body is influenced. It is noteworthy that these reflexes are most easily evoked from the foremost part of the body, from the head, in which the telereceptive sense-organs are situated, so that distance stimuli influencing the position of the head can in this way also impress different attitudes upon the whole body. The attitudinal tonic reflexes evoked from the head appear to be practically indefatigable. In changing the position of the head one performs two different things:

(1) changing the position of the head *in space*, and therefore stimulating the otolithic apparatus,

(2) changing the position of the head *in relation to the body*, therefore flexing or twisting the neck and stimulating the proprioceptors of the deep structures of the neck.

Now the question arises what use the normal animal makes of these reflexes. In adults instantaneous photographs show sometimes postures in agreement with the laws of attitudinal activity . . . movements which seem to be facilitated and strengthened by the preliminary starting posture of the head and body. The mechanism as a whole acts in such a way that the head leads and the body follows. The attitudes impressed upon the body by a certain head position in the decerebrate preparation closely resemble the natural attitudes shown by the intact animal during life. Good pictures and statues give the impression of being natural if the body is represented according to the laws of attitudinal reflexes. The attitudinal reflexes form a group of tonic reactions by which the whole body musculature is integrated for a combined and highly adapted function. The entire body follows the direction assumed by the head, and being very often moved in a certain direction under the influence of the receptive higher sense organs. This provides one of the ways in which the relation of the body to its environment is regulated. It needs only to be briefly mentioned that the different attitudes, with their different distribution of tone and tension in the numerous muscles of the body, are associated with different distributions of reflex irritability over the central nervous system. Therefore, one and the same stimulus may cause quite different reflex reactions according to the different attitudes of the animal at the moment the stimulus is applied.

These anatomical and physiological quotations will show that Alexander differed from established opinion chiefly in the degree of emphasis which he has put on this factor of the head-neck relationship, a factor which, though recognized, has not yet been given widespread practical employment; Alexander (1932) went so far as to term this factor "the primary control". "This primary control depends upon a certain use of the head and neck in relation to the rest of the body."

Correction of Faulty Mechanics in Alexander's Method
In view of this it might be said that Alexander had done nothing very different from the "body mechanics" school, save for his accentuation of the head-neck relationship. His chief contribution, however, lay in the next stage, the stage of "correcting faulty mechanics so that the different structures may be able to work as near to normal as possible".

It is pointed out above that the orthopaedists have found it difficult to eliminate psychological considerations when they come to tackle the question of muscle re-education. "Any posture or movement tends to become implanted in the kinaesthetic sense as a habit; generally it is easier and more comfortable to rest and move with a deformity than against it towards correction," writes Sweet (1939), and, as Sherrington has pointed out, "verbal instruction as to how to correct wrong habits of movement and posture is very difficult". Just how difficult this is was borne out by Fox (1945), in an article dealing with the rehabilitation of American psychoneurotic soldiers who presented symptoms of low back pain.

The type of malposture encountered most commonly was a lordosis with weakness of the lower abdominal muscles resulting in protrusion of the abdomen. There was usually an associated forward slump of the head and shoulders. It was found that the most co-operative of these patients were often unable to assume a correct posture even upon specific request. Both for psychologic and personal reasons it was found advisable to direct therapeutic efforts towards a re-adjustment of the patient's inner conception of himself as an erect individual. The treatment demanded the active co-operation of the patient. The patient is not only given the final goal of "standing straight", but learns to call upon the component muscular activity which will produce the desired result, a point which has been emphasized by F. M. Alexander for many years.

This was also the opinion of Sweet (1939). "Fatigue always caused a child to slump. His teacher of physical education and his parents may be constantly saying: 'Stand up! Sit up! Throw your shoulders back.' A child should not be told to 'stand up' without being taught to do it, any more than he should be ordered to do arithmetic without preliminary instruction in fundamentals."

A similar point is made by Hansson (1945) in his article on "Body Mechanics" for the American Council of Physical Education.

It must be remembered when we are dealing with faulty body mechanics that exercises are not always the answer. It must be realized that every effort to change voluntarily the relative positions of the parts of the body is made through the use of motor habits which are expressed in the body adjustment. To change posture, motor habits must first be changed in the motor pathways in the nervous system. With this change, a different muscular response both for balance and for movement will occur. If proper posture be maintained by conscious effort for a short time, then the exercise of reflex tonus will serve to maintain the proper attitude without the patient requiring to give the matter thought and attention.

Kinaesthetic Re-education

Alexander's account of this situation was to say that it is quite useless
to attempt to change motor habits by direct specific action; such an
attempt he calls "end-gaining". It is quite useless, because our
kinaesthetic sense of ourselves, which permits the faulty pattern to
exist, will not possess the "know-how" of a new manner of use until
there has been a slow and steady kinaesthetic re-education. Any form
of remedial exercise or instruction which ignores the need for such
kinaesthetic re-education is bound to fail—to fail, that is to say, in
the sense that, although there may, of course, be a local specific
success in eradicating particular symptoms, it will not touch the
predisposing faulty pattern of general mechanical use. The reason for
the failure (to quote Sweet again), is that, "any posture or method of
movement tends to become implanted in the kinaesthetic sense as a
habit". Futhermore, the "kinaesthetic equivalent" of a movement—
"the remembered experience of using the muscles which is an
indispensable preliminary to the movement in reality" (Le Vay,
1947)—will govern the total motor response until steps have been
taken to re-educate it.

The kinaesthesia will, in fact, be misleading, said Alexander, just
so long as there is distortion of the head-neck relationship—"the
primary control"—for this, in his opinion, conditions the motor
pattern of the whole organism. Coghill (1929) demonstrated embryo-
logically that motor pathways to a muscle precede in growth the
sensory (proprioceptive) pathways from that muscle; so that it is not
unreasonable to suggest that a motor pattern of activity, which will
reduce the distortion of the "primary control", can be brought about
only by a method which holds in check the effect of the already
existent kinaesthetic sense, until a kinaesthetic awareness of the new
re-directed motor activity has had time to become conscious and
reliable.

Discussing the problem in terms of the golf professional who is
teaching his pupil to "keep his eyes on the ball", Alexander (1932)
wrote:

> He would understand that the difficulty could not be met by any
> such purely specific instruction as telling his pupil to keep his eye
> on the ball, for he would recognize that any "will power" exerted
> by a pupil whose use of himself was already misdirected would be
> exerted in the wrong direction, so that the harder he tried to carry
> out such an instruction and the more he "willed" himself to

succeed, the more his use would be misdirected, and the more likely he would be to take his eyes off the ball. From this he would conclude that he must find some way of teaching his pupil to stop the misdirection of his use, and as he observed that the misdirection began the moment the pupil tried to gain his end and make a good stroke, obviously his first step would be to get the pupil to stop "trying to make a good stroke". It is not the degree of "willing" or "trying", but the way in which the energy is directed that is going to make the "willing" or "trying" effective.

This may appear to be straying a long way from the title of my article: "Anxiety and Muscle Tension". I intimated above that I believe that "worrying" is associated with definite neuromuscular activity, and that the habitual recurrence of it in the psychoneurotic is based on an established motor pattern of activity. I suggested above that in learning to control consciously this maldistributed muscle tension much of the "worrying" will disappear.

We are now in a position to see what is meant by "maldistributed muscle tension". In Alexander's view, maldistribution occurs when muscle activity is not co-ordinated through the proper use of the "primary control". The degree and type of the pattern of maldistribution will vary almost indefinitely, but all cases will have this one factor in common: that until there begins to be a restoration of the proper use of the "primary control", the fundamental basis of the illness will remain, and it is only a question of time until it manifests itself in another symptom of maldistributed tension.

Conscious Inhibition of Maldistributed Tension: Alexander's Method
It remains then to discuss the method employed by Alexander for raising the maldistributed pattern of tension to consciousness, and for laying down an improved pattern. The method, although difficult to describe, is simple in practice, particularly with the help of a teacher. It consists basically in giving the patient a stimulus which would, if he reacted to it, "touch off" the maldistributed pattern of motor activity. The patient is, in effect, given an "anxiety", and is then taught not to react to it in a way which involves making tension. Alexander teaches the patient to inhibit his immediate response to this anxiety—that is to refuse to give immediate expression to the old "kinaesthetic equivalent" which is evoked by the particular stimulus —and instead to project consciously a new pattern of activity. To this end the patient is assisted by a teacher, who will indicate just in what respects the patient's response to the stimulus manifests itself

in maldistribution of muscle tension; in this way, very slowly, a new awareness of his manner of using himself is gradually built up, until he becomes more and more proficient in controlling his reactions. The severity of the stimulus—the "anxiety"—can be gradually increased, whilst the patient acquires more and more confidence in preserving a stable response under such circumstances. This may take weeks or months but, if it is persisted in, it will be found that the confidence gained in this way will be transferred into other situations. As Bernard Shaw (1937) said: "Alexander has established not only the beginning of a far-reaching science of the apparently involuntary movements we call reflexes, but a technique of correction and self-control which forms a substantial addition to our very slender resources in personal education."

It may be that Alexander has, indeed, come upon a fundamental truth about man's inheritance as an organism—a truth which would go far towards lessening the unhappiness of modern civilization. Only time, and the repeated careful utilization of his method, can give the answer to this.

ELEVEN

Alexander's View of Psychoanalysis
by Marjory Alexander Barlow

ALTHOUGH FREUD AND Alexander were almost exact contemporaries, it is unlikely that Alexander came in contact with Freudian ideas until after his own discoveries had been made and his own working procedures well established. He was, on first principles, opposed to the idea of psychoanalysis since it implied division, and an approach to human difficulties from the psychological angle only. He believed that a human being functioned as a whole and could only be fundamentally changed as a whole.

The term psychophysical is used throughout my works [he wrote], to indicate the impossibility of separating physical and mental processes in the working of the human organism. . . . Psychoanalysis is based on the same specific "end-gaining" principle as the methods which it is claimed by some to supersede. Take the case of a person who suffers from some unreasoning fear, and goes to a psychoanalyst for help. Supposing he and the analyst together unravel the knot and decide that the origin of the fear lies in some event or train of events which took place in the past and unduly excited the patient's fear reflexes, and established a phobia.

I have pointed out that all so-called mental activity is a process governed by our psychophysical condition at the time when the particular stimulus is received. A person falls into some unreasoning fear because his condition of psychophysical functioning at the time when he receives the stimulus is unsatisfactory. He must have been beset at this time with imperfect co-ordination, imperfect adjustment, and unreliable and delusive sensory appreciation. What can be done by the unravelling procedure of psychoanalysis to remedy these serious defects of general psychophysical functioning? Will psychoanalysis as practised restore a reliable sensory appreciation to the patient, and co-ordinate and re-educate his psychophysical mechanisms on a general basis? Certainly not. The psychophysical condition which permitted the establishment of the first phobia will permit the establishment of another. The method of psychoanalysis is another instance of the "end-gaining" attempt to effect the "cure" of a specific trouble by specific means without consideration being given to the necessity of restoring a satisfactory standard of psychophysical functioning.

Psychoanalysis has, of course, moved a long way since Alexander wrote about it. Its procedures in this country are now more concerned with interpersonal relations and a person's reactions to his own internal stimuli. It is probable that this later development would have been more to Alexander's liking, since his own work fore-shadowed this development in its emphasis on the need to become aware of internal reaction. However, his objection to the "partial" nature of the psychoanalytical remedy would still stand.

Before we can make any real attempt to reach a satisfactory state of awareness—that is, to know ourselves—we must reach a satis-factory state of co-ordination and we must employ this in every act of daily life.... Comparatively few of us recognize that our manner of use has anything to do with the nature of our func-tioning or of our reaction to stimuli; nor the extent to which our physical-mental well-being depends upon the manner in which we use ourselves during our waking and sleeping hours.... The majority of people have developed a manner of use of themselves which is constantly exerting a harmful influence not only upon their functioning but also upon their manner of reaction. We should be able to see that this wrong use can be a source of indivi-dual failings, peculiarities, wrong ideas and ills of all kinds, as well as of that inward unrest and unhappiness which is evident in the social life of to-day.

Psychophyscial Happiness

This last quotation shows how much Alexander was concerned with the absence of real happiness manifested by the majority of adults today, and he attributed this to the fact that they are experiencing a continually deteriorating use of themselves, setting up conditions of physical irritation and pressure.

"Irritation" was a favourite word with Alexander and he meant by it the restlessness, muscular agitation and quick "irritability" of emotional reaction that seem to characterize so many people today.

Small wonder that under these conditions the person concerned becomes more and more irritated and unhappy. Every effort made by someone who is already in an irritated condition will tend to make him still more irritated, and therefore as time goes on his chances of happiness diminish. Furthermore, his experiences of happiness become of even shorter duration, until at last he is forced to take refuge in a state of unhappiness and depression, in which his reasoning is in abeyance and he is dominated by his emotional impulses. . . . Such a person will be irritated by experiences which would not have the least effect on one whose sensory appreciation is reliable.

Subconscious Habit

The term "unconscious" does not appear in Alexander's early writings except by implication, in that his basic thesis was the need to develop consciousness. "Man's success in developing his potentialities . . . will depend upon whether or not he can reach a plane of living where he substitutes conscious guidance and control of the use of himself for the instinctive (automatic) self guidance and control."

He wrote a great deal about subconscious habit:

Subconsciousness is only a synonym for that rigid routine we refer to as habit—this rigid routine being the stumbling-block to rapid adaptability and to the assimilation of new ideas, to originality. On the other hand, consciousness is the synonym for mobility of mind, mobility which subconscious control checks and impedes, mobility which will obtain for us physical regeneration and the wider enjoyment of those powers which we all possess but which are often deliberately stunted or neglected.

With all of this, no doubt, the analyst would agree. Any divergence there might be would be over the means of obtaining this desirable state.

It was Alexander's claim that so long as there was subjection of muscular habits to subconscious control, fixed habits of thought could not be eliminated. "What is called for is a fundamental change in the use of the self by means of which the standard of functioning will be raised and psychophysical defects and ills, whether fears or any other emotional reactions, will be overcome." Above all he held that "the conscious mind must be quickened". He was not optimistic that analysis alone would do this in a lasting and fundamental manner, and such is the subtlety of the actual practical procedures which he evolved, that much of what the analyst seeks to do is, in fact, carried out in the Alexander "lesson". The need to "work through" a depression becomes a reality when the teacher himself is able to

E

give the pupil the actual experience of "non-depression". Certainly this experience is not at a verbal level, but many would say that it is at a level deeper than verbal communication. The rapport which is established with the Alexander teacher by such experiences can, and often does, lead on to an unburdening of basic worries and anxieties.

Alexander knew well that his work was only a beginning and he made it quite clear that he did not profess to offer a finally perfected method. It is to be hoped that with an increasing number of psychiatrists and analysts taking an interest in the Alexander approach, a fruitful pooling of resources can take place.

TWELVE

Jung and Alexander: The Common Ground
by Dr Nina Meyer

JUNG IS DESCRIBED by J. B. Priestley in his essays on contemporary events as "not only one of the greatest original thinkers of our times, but also one of its few liberators". How does Jung play his part in this liberation of functioning? To understand this it is necessary to outline three of his important concepts, which are especially relevant to the relationship of Jung and Alexander. Both Jung and Alexander were concerned, from different standpoints, with essentially the same matter, that is, with whole and healthy functioning.

These three concepts are those of the Self, the Archetypes, and, standing between them, Jung's definition of the Ego. Let us see what he says of each of them: first, the Ego, since this is the uniting bridge between Self and Archetype, and this is the concept perhaps easiest to place within the structure of Alexander's teaching.

The Ego

"Experience shows", says Jung, "that the Ego rests on two seemingly different bases, the somatic and the psychic. The somatic is produced by endosomatic stimuli, only some of which cross the threshold of consciousness. A considerable proportion of these stimuli occur unconsciously." Included amongst these endosomatic stimuli are, of course, the kinaesthetic stimuli which Alexander describes.

"The somatic basis of the Ego", Jung continues, "consists of conscious and unconscious factors. The same is true of the psychic basis. The Ego seems to arise in the first place from the collision between the somatic factor and the environment, and once established, it goes on developing from the further collisions with the outer world and the inner."

Jung's recognition of the part played by endosomatic factors in Egoformation has its counterpart in Alexander's account of the manner in which kinaesthetic sensibility may be distorted and submerged by the impact of the environment, leading to the setting up of muscular habits which may be irrelevant and useless as well as those which may be relevant and useful in the conscious day-to-day life. What Alexander describes as "end-gaining" appears to be a manifestation of the Ego as described by Jung. And Jung's idea of the

Ego arising from the collision of the "somatic factor" and environment also postulates that "the term psychic be used only where there is evidence of a will capable of modifying reflex or instinctual processes". This would also appear to link up closely with Alexander's concept of the use of inhibition to modulate reflex end-gaining reactions.

The Archetypes

How does this lead on to the theme of the Archetypes and of the Self? First, the Archetypes: much has been written about this difficult theme by Jung and also by students of his work. In trying to put it simply, I would say that the Archetype is a potential for experience, a readiness to respond to stimuli with certain kinds of imagery, which are related to constitutional or inborn patterns, and that such imagery in turn influences thought and behaviour. How does Jung put it? He says:

> The psychological manifestations of the instincts I have termed Archetypes: they are living entities which cause the preformation of numinous ideas or dominant representations. They become manifest in the ever-recurring patterns of psychic functioning. Man, despite his freedom and superficial changeability, will function psychologically according to his original patterns—up to a certain point; that is, until for some reason he collides with his still-living and ever-present instinctual roots. The instincts will then protest and engender peculiarly shaped thoughts and emotions.

Whilst Alexander would probably not agree with Jung's concept of Instinct, it would appear that the basic Alexander tenet of "total pattern response" is very close to Jung's idea of an Archetype. It is the goal of Alexander's re-education to restore contact with this "total pattern reaction", based as it is on a "normal" neuromuscular sequence of response which travels cephalo-caudad unless interfered with. And the collision with ever-present instinctual roots, which cause "peculiarly shaped thoughts and emotions", and which result in symptoms and neurotic patternings, will therefore be manifested in disturbances of postural and distortion of the total pattern of reaction.

It seems to me that Alexander was trying to liberate these still-living instinctual roots by his method of inhibiting those responses that prevent the freely flowing libido from being given expression during the confrontation of the "somatic factor" with the environment. This contact with instinctual roots seems to me to be the meaning also of Zen philosophy, which is so near to Alexander's teaching. This psychosomatic unity has been enlarged on by Dr Barlow, and it is in this context that I have tried to put something of Jung's concept before you. In Jung's definition of the Self, this becomes even clearer.

The Self

It is here, however, that definitions are most difficult—perhaps because Jung, unlike Freud, was not convinced of the power of words. For Freud, "words and magic were in the beginning one and the same thing". For Jung, on the other hand, "the image is the preliminary stage of the idea—its maternal soil". He says: "Our intellect is born from mythology, and mythology is nothing but a translation of inner experience into the language of pictures and speech, which is a storehouse of images founded on experience."

In this emphasis on experience, Jung and Alexander have much in common, and this is particularly so in the sphere of the Self which, for Jung, is a psychological concept to account for the experience of completeness and totality. As Jung puts it, "Although 'wholeness' seems at first sight to be nothing but an abstract idea, it is nevertheless empirical insofar as it is anticipated by the psyche in the form of spontaneous symbols. Their significance as symbols of unity and totality is amply confirmed by empirical psychology, something that exists and can be experienced." For Jung, the greatest significance of the Self is as an integrating process most apparent in adult life; and it is closely bound up with his therapeutic teaching.

These concepts have been developed by what we can call the Neo-Jungian school of his pupils. For Neuman, "the Self is the original state of totality out of which the individual Ego is born"; and Fordham, on the basis of clinical observation of infants and children, also postulates the Self as the original totality prior to the emergence of the Ego. For me, its application has been most important in the development of the child, and particularly in the mother-child relationship; the observation of the manifold physical expressions of the earliest mother-child interaction has been of the greatest help in my work as a psychiatrist in neo-natal and infant welfare clinics. It is here that I have found my acquaintance with Alexander's teaching most helpful.

It will be seen from this that there is some overlap in Alexander's concept of the total pattern and the Jungian concept of the Self.

Both perhaps would agree that the Self is a term which encompasses the wholeness of experience, though Alexander might use the term to include the neuro-muscular basis of interpersonal relationship.

It is impossible in a brief survey such as this to do more than touch on some basic Jungian concepts. This description of Jung as a liberator of our time is embodied in the present psychiatric view of disturbances of functioning as disturbances in the psycho-soma of the Self. It is here that Jung and Alexander seem to me to come together as two aspects of a unitary functioning.

THIRTEEN

The Process of Growth
by Dr Robin Skynner

(An address given at the Alexander Institute in 1967 during
a symposium on the psychological aspects of Alexander's work)

ALL GROWTH AND development takes place by discontinuous
steps, in which periods of temporary disintegration are followed by
reintegration at a new and higher level. In development of motor
skills, the child passes through definite phases in which his motor
patterns are co-ordinated and secure. Each of these is followed by a
period of clumsiness and uncertainty, where the pattern seems temporarily to be lost, before a new level of organization is reached,
more complex than the old.

Similarly, the child's psychological development, phases of
disequilibrium and lack of confidence occur between each successive
phase of increased stability and assurance. It cannot be otherwise,
since a pattern must be dismantled, at least to some extent, and then
reassembled, if basic improvements are to be made. Gesell and his
followers have traced this physical and psychological ebb and flow
in the growth of children in fascinating detail.

Though more readily observable in the rapid changes occurring in
the young, this law that new and improved patterns can only arise
from the temporary breakdown and apparent loss of the pre-existing
ones probably applies to any form of growth and development, no
matter at what age this occurs. However, we are particularly blind and
resistant to the operation of this law in ourselves. We always seek to
add to our stature, to improve on what we are already, to keep the
security of what we have while reaching out for change. Yet the
more fundamental the impending change, the more it must feel to us
like a threatened dissolution and loss of everything that really matters
in us, everything we most essentially feel we *are*.

My second point is that the physical and psychological growth of
children takes place by a limiting of the rich diversity of possibilities
present in the embryo. We develop *this* attitude rather than *that* one,
feel we are this kind of person rather than another, prefer "good" to
"evil" or "evil" to "good". Organization takes place at the cost of

restriction of the potentialities of the personality, or in other terms, at the cost of repression and the division into two categories of psychic contents, conscious and unconscious, one category containing all we think we are and the other all we think we are not.

Though growth of this kind continues throughout life, new demands and stresses calling for new adaptations, most people remain more or less satisfied with what they have become. Others, probably a small proportion but larger perhaps than one suspects, never lose the feeling that they have lost something in the process of growing up, and seek to regain a dimly felt state of completeness and harmony that once existed. These people will tend to seek out systems and techniques that can aid them in the rediscovery of what they have lost, and extending the "conscious self" to include within its organization these once repressed contents of the larger, total "self". The part, once extruded from the whole and subjected to a necessary process of development, now seeks to reunite with it and take back with it what it has learned. I suggest that many kinds of aid exist to facilitate this process of rediscovery. Among others, I mention specifically the Alexander Technique and depth techniques in psychotherapy (whether Freudian, Jungian or any other) and the great religions including Christianity, as meeting this wish for rediscovery of the self on different levels and scales.

My third point is really a fusion of these two previous ones. All prospect of growth creates an ambivalent attitude within us. We yearn for some extension of ourselves, yet fear the dissolution of ourselves that first has to occur. Part of us wishes to proceed to the next step on the staircase, while part clings to the security of the step we know and stand on since the change has, by its nature, to take place without foreknowledge of the result.

Now my main thesis is that any system that can be used to facilitate an extension of the existing personality can also be used to prevent such a development, and that it is precisely where a system is most powerful to aid us that it can also be used most effectively to block our progress. We see this on the biggest scale in the transmission of religious systems, where what begins as an attempt to break down existing prejudices and habits of experience becomes in the course of time a new dogma, the supporters of which persecute the new saint who threatens to upset the *status quo* by throwing everything open to question again and offering, not comfort and security, but "rebirth". The Christian seeks to be better, instead of seeking to know what he is and to be given the strength to bear it.

On the smaller scale of psychological treatment, the analyst discovers that the understanding which enables him to help others proves the biggest obstacle to his obtaining help for himself. The techniques with which he exposes his patients to the immediate experiences they fear and avoid can be used by him as a new and more efficient form of avoidance, interposing thought and theory between himself and his life.

Each system, I have suggested, has its most central and effective principle, which can be used for or against its aim. The Alexander Technique can be no exception, and I leave it as a question for the audience what the most specific form of *mis*use of the Technique can be, suggesting only that, by analogy with other systems, it will probably be so subtly close to its proper use as to be almost indistinguishable.

Of course, use and misuse are themselves perhaps relative terms. It may be that what is appropriate "use" in a phase of vulnerability and disintegration would be misuse in the ensuing period of reconstruction and consolidation, and that we need to know what to use at the right time. Certainly control and safety, at the expense of expansion and widening of the personality, among some who use the Technique, appears to be the main reason for some anatagonism to the methods of depth psychology—some of whose adherents tend to err equally, but in the opposite direction.

The answer? I have my own, at least for the moment, but as soon as we feel we have *the* answer we are stuck again. So I leave it open for you as for myself.

FOURTEEN

Hide or Seek
by Dorothea Wallis

THE ALEXANDER TECHNIQUE is designed to teach one to use one's body rationally and economically instead of unconsciously and inappropriately. It teaches the basic principle that there is a particular state or "body-scheme" in which the parts of the body are so related and muscular tension is so distributed that each part and the whole is enabled to be and to function at its best.

Alexander came to define this scheme by patient, concentrated self-observation, by finding out where the misuse of himself led to inefficiency and then freeing himself of his "bad old ways" by deliberately directing himself according to the rational scheme that made for the most effective manner of use. His personal achievement in doing this led him to assume that to apply his technique was specifically a matter of conscious thought and control.

However important the part of conscious thought and control in the Alexander Technique, they are only aspects of a whole personality and not independent entities. To treat them as such, and ignore the whole of which they are a limited aspect, would be to impair any process of re-education; for education is a matter of the whole personality. Alexander's emphasis on the unity of body and mind recognizes this, but his claim needs to be substantiated by a fuller understanding of the kind of changes his process of re-education involves in terms other than the strictly physical in which he himself gives a detailed account.

In "physical terms" it may be said that a central theme of the Alexander Technique is to learn to inhibit one's usual reaction to any stimulus, and by ordering oneself into a relatively balanced position to react deliberately with only a suitable kind and amount of tension. When I hear the door bell ring, I may habitually be shocked into an apprehensive state of overall tension. According to Alexander's teaching I try to inhibit this reaction of my neck and head as the centre of control, direct it into a freer state and, having reduced my state of irrelevant tension, walk to the door. These physical changes may be an observable fact, but such an account of what happens seems to me so inadequate as not to be a description of a real person or real event at all. It is a kind of theoretical construction which bears little resemblance to reality. It is as informative a description of myself and my reaction to the door bell as a purely statistical description of a group of people is of their character as individuals and their relationships to each other.

The apparently simple incident of a bell ringing and my going to answer it, far from being a single incident—with a simple "stimulus-response" pattern—is one thread in a closely knit complex of time and place, myself, my past and expectations. A single stimulus may be a useful idea, but does not exist in normal life (if ever even in experimental conditions) just as "a bell" can never ring. If one is to understand what the Alexander Technique tries to do, it seems essential to recognize this. The idea of a single stimulus and response seems to me as much an obstacle in the way of understanding the technique as in other ways it may be a help. It is an obstacle because it makes incomprehensible the state of general tension in which I may normally go to the door when the bell rings. This can be understood when, instead of the bell being thought of as "a stimulus" and my reaction as "a response", they are seen in their particular context as details of a total personal world. Superfluous tension in one's behaviour is obviously not due only to poor judgement of what is demanded of one by the physical environment. The way in which one uses one's body is as much a response to one's mental as to one's physical situation. To change one's response to the inner situation may be far more difficult than changing one's reaction to the external world. It is much harder to admit feeling very small and vulnerable inside, but decide not to stand huddled up and speak in an evasive way as one is accustomed to do, than it is to make the adjustment which is necessary when one goes from a steep to a shallow flight of steps.

To learn the Alexander Technique is a formidable task because the change in the use of one's body demands such drastic mental reorientation. I don't think the physical change can be made, except temporarily, without the mental reorientation. What does this reorientation amount to? The Alexander Technique gives me an objective standard for a sound way of using my body. If I adopt this impersonal standard instead of a habitual personal one, I stand and move in a way I consider suitable rather than the way I happen to feel like. If I feel like being crumpled up because I am miserable but refuse to let my feeling determine the way I actually sit or stand, and in fact stand freely, can it be said that I am disguising or suppressing my real feelings by an insincere pose? On the contrary, to refuse to let an emotion govern the behaviour of one's body is not to suppress it but to refuse it an effective disguise, and this in turn means that one has to face it.

What light does this throw on the particular case in which I try to apply the Alexander Technique, of answering the door bell? The sound of the door bell puts me into a state of anxious apprehension and tension. I normally go to open the door in this tense, "tight" state. Applying the technique, I stop for a moment and consciously direct my head, neck, etc., into a freer state before I walk to the door. In trying to free myself from the excessive tension, I am trying to free my body and behaviour from being dominated by an objectively irrelevant feeling.

In doing this I am perhaps no nearer to knowing just what I fear at the sound of the door bell, but I become more clearly aware of the existence of this feeling of fear which has nothing to do with the present situation but has a persistent influence on me. It not only is irrelevant to the present situation, but is an encumbrance which prevents me from being alert and adaptable to the present. I believe that some such recognition, even though it may be inarticulate, of the feeling that is the motive force of the tension I try to undo, is an essential part of the release of that tension.

The importance of this step is a kind of separation of one's self— an independent conscious part—from deeply grounded emotional attitudes. To find out the feeling that is behind the tension does not mean getting rid of it. In the example of the door bell, I take my fear with me when I go to the door, but don't let it go for me. In this way one may be able to separate the emotional patterns which dominate one through resolving the tensions they make; they are not put *away*, but put into their proper place and no longer allowed freely to take possession of one. Is this process comparable to the cure of a neurosis in which a part of oneself that has become autonomous is deprived of its excessive power?

This sort of reorganization is not made by regulating one's body once or a few times according to a new conscious pattern. Probably only by persistent, laborious working at this does one reach the emotional background of the tensions one tries to change. But perhaps only in arriving and tackling the situation at this level does the Alexander Technique become a process of re-education. It seems to me that without this it would produce only momentary changes which could not be maintained.

Unfortunately, one's excessive tensions are not produced by one single emotional force which once discovered can be put out of action. One probably can point to one source of all undue tension, a basic insecurity of the personality, but this rather than being one feeling is a condition, more or less unchanging, from which grow the many different emotional attitudes which produce tension. To apply the Alexander Technique seems to be an endless task of meeting and disarming these many different attitudes rather than drastically discovering one "dragon" and staging a valiant fight to free oneself from it. The one emotional cause—which has been called ontological or existential insecurity—is a fundamental state like being very tall or small. One cannot alter one's tallness, but if it makes one stoop one can stop stooping and admit one's size. Similarly, one probably cannot help being insecure but if it makes one afraid and hesitant, or aggressive at every turn and correspondingly "knotted-up" and tense, one can perhaps by resolving the physical tension stop taking the fears at their face value and recognize their underlying cause. The insecurity, like the tallness, remains, but one can come to live with it rather than for it.

This ultimate source of tension may be recognized implicitly in Alexander's concept of "end-gaining", as the evil his technique is intended to counteract. He urges that in whatever we do, whether getting out of a chair or hitting a golf ball, we must concentrate on the "means-whereby" rather than the end. What do we do when we are "end-gaining"—which undoubtedly we do a lot of the time, from working for the "eleven plus" to making the right conversation at a party? We are not so much concerned with what we are doing as with how we show up. When Alexander's player is intent only on his ball rather than the way he deals with it, his anxiety is to prove himself the good player that he needs to be to satisfy himself. When the housewife strenuously scrubs her kitchen floor the strain comes from trying to live up to her own high standards rather than the difficulty of the job.

The "end" in "end-gaining" is always to reinforce a weak self. "End-gaining" is characteristic of the insecure person—which perhaps most of us are to a greater or lesser degree—who finds it necessary to look for confirmation of himself in whatever he does. To be "end-gaining" means to use oneself with excessive tension. The tension arises from the effort of justifying or proving oneself in the world instead of simply being part of it. If one can be in oneself and not forever reaching out to make up for what one is not, then one can do things for their own sake and does not "end-gain". In the end, Alexander's standard for the balanced regulation of the body, to be and work at its best, is the standard of a whole, sound person.

FIFTEEN

The Deeper Significance of Posture and Movement
by Dr Grahame Fagg

TO ME TRUTH is like a rope made of a number of strands. It should be possible to follow a different facet of the truth along its own strand. A different view does not invalidate the others but in fact may strengthen them. Before my physical experiences with the Alexander Principle I had taken many of my psychological beliefs on trust. This new experience has confirmed some and made me question others.

Mimicry

The advantages of being a paediatrician are many. I can see my patients in the nude without causing embarrassment and also I see them with their families, and this has confirmed the tremendous force of mimicry. It is in the toddler period that children copy their parents, and this is so important a factor in their behaviour later on that if, as parents, the behaviour of our children is annoying then they are almost certainly copying us—not necessarily as we are now, but as we were when they were toddlers.

When I started Alexander lessons I was also practising as a paediatrician and I started straight away trying things out on my patients. I soon discovered that I was imprinting my own faults of posture and movement on them. They were becoming mirrors of myself and as such were of great value to me when I realized what was happening. Apart from this however I found that I was catching behaviour from them, and of course this is so in all human contact—in fact in all contact between living things. Married couples grow like each other, the dog behaves like his master, who in turn becomes like his dog!

Chronic Emotional States

After mimicry as a factor moulding human behaviour comes the adoption of fixed postures which show (and perpetuate) chronic emotional states. Just as the acute emotion always produces its temporary facial expression and bodily posture which automatically affects breathing speech and movement, so the chronic emotional imbalance leads to persistently distorted posture and movement.

In handling children it soon became apparent that there were two situations. The one in which the chronic emotional state is still active and alight—the other in which the passion is spent, the fire dead. In this second situation it is easy to re-educate with great relief to the person concerned—in the first situation it is difficult to help. Exactly the same situation occurs in asthma. Allergy, infection or emotion may produce asthma with its typical breathing pattern and muscle tensions. The original cause may pass but the asthma be perpetuated by the habit patterns. At this stage it is easy to help the asthmatic by the physical approach.

Debility
After mimicry and chronic emotional states there is another important element in posture in children and this is the drooping debilitated state which we see so often, and I wonder whether we do enough to rehabilitate people after a period of illness. They cannot be left automatically to recover especially if they return to the fray too soon.

Conditioned Reflexes
The factors already mentioned tend to produce stereotyped behaviour in the person which is present all the time, while children who have learned certain skills under emotional stress may show the same emotion in their posture whenever they perform that activity, be it walking or talking, reading or writing or some passive situation such as having a hair-cut. The strange thing is that when there is no longer a strong emotion associated with the situation, the habit pattern of behaviour will tend to generate or recreate that emotion.

Behaviour of Particular Age Groups
The real strength of the paediatrician's position is that he gets to know the typical behaviour of a child at different ages from infancy to adult life, and he can therefore spot at once behaviour which is wrong for the person's age—and this is usually behaviour belonging to an earlier age. This behaviour can be taken as an indication that there has been a block in normal development at that age and if one can take the subject back to that point he may well be helped to overcome unsolved difficulties. The psychoanalysts work on this principle and make very heavy weather of it. Not only does a study of physical behaviour help us to pinpoint the probable age of trouble quickly, but using physical experiences to recall the past can produce considerable emotional reactions with beneficial results.

Going through typical physical behaviour by age groups we start with the first three months of life, when the important factor is lack of head control—the head having to be managed by the mother—and what is the main activity of the Alexander teacher? Also in this age he characteristically fixes his mother's face with an unblinking gaze.

At four months he has head control—he smiles at all faces, strange or familiar, he takes pleasure in his own voice and finds his own hands fascinating to play with.

At seven months he is sitting with a back shaped in a single curve from neck to sacrum. He explores his environment with his eyes. He experiences new tastes and consistencies of food. He lies awake and meditates for hours on end. How many of us return to this age on holiday or in the evening of life?

At last he becomes mobile—he crawls; he stands; he walks and he explores, but he must always have the security of his mother close at hand. He has pain with teething. He learns to speak and to recognize pictures and symbols in books. At first he has no fear but then he learns to know danger.

Later, at three years he moves away from his dependence on his mother and is ready to enter the nursery group. He has in this toddler stage been prone to rages as a response to frustration, and when mixing with children of his own age he will indulge in fights for what he wants.

At four years he starts to ask "what's that" and at five he asks "Why?" so his parents send him to school! He starts to learn the three Rs. At this age he commonly develops the hate posture of lifted shoulders and tightened neck—the boxer's posture.

Fear—Hate

We can of course explain all as a matter of repressed aggression, and the tight neck and hunched shoulders express a particular form of aggression—that of the child against authority. The reciprocal of this is the stiffening up and the tucking in of the chin—the caricature of the judge or the elderly schoolmistress. This is the aggressive posture of authority towards the underdog—the adult towards the child.

There is a similar pelvic posture of fear and aggression and it is interesting to note that there is always a distortion of posture in both the neck, shoulder and pelvic regions. One cannot have a normal lumbar, pelvic and hip posture with distortion in the neck and shoulder, nor can one have the reverse.

The Significance of Parts of the Body

I come now to a more fanciful method of interpreting posture, and especially of body tensions. Suppose we could determine the basic significance of certain parts of the body, then tensions between different parts might indicate conflicts between the forces symbolized by these parts of the body, and more simply the exaggeration of these parts of the body would have a positive significance, either suggesting that the personality of the person is exaggerated in this way or, more likely, that there has been a block in expression and the person is perpetuating and exaggerating a certain form of posture because this facet of the personality has not been allowed to be expressed for social or other reasons.

Take firstly the two main areas of tension in the back, they are the neck and the lumbar region and of course these are the two mobile parts of the spine coming between the thoraco-abdominal region on the one hand and the head above and the pelvis below. It seems to me that the self is situated in the chest and abdomen. Authority; society; parents; teachers; church; law; medicine; superego—reside in the head; Alexander was right in putting neck tensions first. Most of our troubles stem from conflict with society and with parents, who see themselves as society's main agents in their dealings with the toddler.

This conflict between self and society generates within us a sense of right and wrong, as appreciated by the toddler, and we cast out the evil into the pelvis, that sink of iniquity to do with sex and lavatories. So we get a false division of the body in motion and instead of bending at our hip joints, those beautiful ball and socket joints made for free movement, we bend in the lumbar spine which is meant to move much less. So the devil resides in the pelvis; he did not always do so—in fact he did not always exist. You will remember he is a fallen angel, our unwanted past. He is in fact two devils—the one a genuine devil cast out by GOD—truly unwanted, the other a much larger one, grey rather than black and cast out by society. So the conflict between head and body generates the conflict between body and pelvis. As we mature we colonize our heads and eliminate some of the conflict and the Alexander teacher helps to speed the process.

Another area of tension in the back is the lower thoracic region. Is this the battlefield between chest and abdomen, and if so what do these parts of the torso mean?

The chest is where the spirit resides—life itself. When, as animals in the distant past, our ancestors first became aware of life and death, it was breathing which was of significance and those of us who have witnessed death are aware of the shrinking of the chest which occurs at that moment. Expiration and expiry are the same thing. With each breathing cycle we approach death and regain life again. Those with most vitality tend to have expanded chests, but also those who fear death may over expand to keep further away from that which they fear.

The chest is moving, active, male, the abdomen passive, female. Are tensions in the lower dorsal region evidence of the conflict between the male and the female within us, the projected conflicts between our parents?

So we can speculate on the significance of posture and can read many messages which are written clearly while others may be in code and we cannot be absolutely certain of their meaning.

APPLICATIONS

THEOLOGICAL

SIXTEEN

End-Gaining and Means-Whereby
by Aldous Huxley

PREACHING IS ONE of the major professions and one of the commonest of hobbies. Perhaps a tenth of the entire human race spends all or part of its time telling the other nine-tenths what ends they should pursue, and how they should act, think, and feel, in order to please God, remain healthy, get on in the world, and promote the welfare of the community. Some of this advice is definitely pernicious; but most of it is sound enough, and not a little of it is in accord with the highest ethical and religious idealism.

What is the effect of all this education, first, upon those preached to, and, second, upon the preachers? The headlines in the newspapers provide a horribly depressing answer to the first question. The answer to the second is hardly less dismal; for if we read the biographies of defunct idealists, if we cultivate the acquaintance of those most busily engaged in telling what they ought to do to be saved, physically, morally, politically, and spiritually, we shall find that very many preachers conspicuously fail to practise what they preach. We shall meet with philosophers whose lives are hopelessly irrational and mean; religious leaders at the mercy of their passions and prejudices; physicians ignoring their own rules of health and living in chronically diseased bodies; politicians whose conduct, in the affairs of State, is frankly criminal; professional educators conducting themselves with the vanity and silliness of children. The tree is known by its fruits, and from a study of the fruits of preaching it is evident that something is decidedly wrong with that particular tree.

We have a direct intuition of the value of the highest moral and religious ideals; and we know empirically that the accepted methods of inculcating those ideals are not very effective. Politicians may embark on large-scale social reforms, designed to improve the world, but these reforms cannot produce more than a fraction of the good results expected of them, unless educators discover means whereby preachers and preached-to can implement their good intentions and practise what is preached. To build this bridge between idealistic theory and actual practice has proved so difficult that most men and women have hitherto merely evaded the problem. For either they have gone on preaching and teaching as in the past, regardless of the fact that the old educational methods are only about ten per cent efficient. Or else, having realized that the gap between theory and practice is still unbridged, they have turned against the preachers and even the ideals preached by them. Regardless of the fact that cynicism and blind fanaticism are equally disastrous, they have become moral and intellectual nihilists, and, from nihilism, have gone on, under the spell of some fascinating demagogue, to the service of one of the idolatrous pseudo-religions such as nationalism, fascism, or communism. Meanwhile, the original problem remains unsolved and the circumstances of the time become less and less favourable to the rational solution of any social or psychological problem whatsoever.

Up to the present time only two solutions have been discovered to the problem of bridging the gap between idealistic theory and actual practice. The first, which is very ancient, is the mystic's technique of transcending personality in a progressive awareness of ultimate reality. The second, which is very recent, was discovered some 50 years ago by F. M. Alexander and may be described as a technique for the proper use of the self, a method for the creative conscious control of the whole psychophysical organism.

Alexander's fundamental discovery was this: there exists in man, as in all the other vertebrates, a primary control conditioning the proper use of the total organism. When the head is in a certain relation to the neck, and the neck in a certain relation to the trunk, then (it is a matter of brute empirical fact) the entire psychophysical organism is functioning to the best of its natural capacity. When, for any reason whatsoever, the proper relations between head, neck, and trunk are disturbed, the psychophysical organism comes to be used improperly.

Animals in the state of nature and human beings in primitive conditions rely on instinct to keep the mechanism of the primary control working as it ought to work. But, with the rise of civilization, environment begins to change with increasing rapidity. Human beings find themselves continually called upon to adapt themselves to unfamiliar circumstances. They become disturbed, and their bewilderment interferes with their instincts, with the result that the primary control ceases to be exercised and the self comes to be improperly used. Improper use of the self produces physical and mental conditions which call urgently for cure and reform. But all attempts at cure and reform are now doomed to more or less complete insuccess. For so long as their own and their neighbour's primary control remains faulty, all that even the best-intentioned reformers can do for themselves and other people cannot in the nature of things result in anything but the perpetuation and perhaps the intensification of the prevailing improper use of the self.

We are all, in Alexander's phrase, "end-gainers". We have goals towards which we hasten without ever considering the means whereby we, as psychophysical organisms, can best achieve our purpose. Most education is strictly of the end-gaining kind. We urge our children towards the goals of knowledge, morality, and health, without instructing them in the proper use of the psychophysical organisms which are to acquire these goals. The consequence is that the goals are acquired imperfectly and at a high price in terms of malfunctioning. Some educators, it is true, pay attention to the "means-whereby", but unfortunately they know nothing of the primary control which insures the proper use of the self. In their ignorance, they try to eliminate defects and establish improvements by a process of direct attack. But such direct attacks cannot, in the nature of things, be effective. True, bad symptoms may be palliated by direct methods and a measure of partial good achieved, but these results are always obtained at a high price. For, if the primary control is faulty, all intensive activity, however well intentioned and whatever the partial improvements achieved, can only help to ingrain the habits of improper use. This means that any good achieved will be accompanied by harmful by-products, which may actually outweigh it, if not immediately, then in the long run. In all that concerns life, it is only through the indirect approach that the most substantial goods are achieved. Thus religion is valueless when it seeks the immediate advantage of the devotee. To the mystic it is axiomatic that he must seek first the kingdom of God and His righteousness. Similarly, the moralist perceives that happiness is not achieved by the direct pursuit of happiness. Happiness is a by-product, the result of pursuing other ends than happiness, by other than merely pleasurable means. In the same way, the complete correction of bad physical or mental habits is not to be achieved by treatments or exercises designed to palliate the specific bodily symptoms, nor by acts of will designed to change the undesirable patterns of thought and behaviour, but only indirectly, through learning to master the the primary control of the organism as a whole.

The technique of mastering the primary control can be learnt unaided, as Alexander learnt it before his looking-glass, 50 years ago. But the difficulties in the way of self-education are so great that the vast majority of individuals will find it quite impossible to inhibit the tendencies to bad habits of use, and to acquire good habits, without the aid of an experienced teacher. At the present time there exist in the world only a few dozens of such teachers. Alexander has had to do his work of training almost single-handed and without any official support. Those who control the educational machine ignore his discovery. Instead of working to make available to all this newly discovered bridge between idealistic theory and actual practice, they waste their own and their pupils' time in carrying out crusades for Liberal Education, Modern Education, Scientific Education, or whatever it may be, in selecting the Hundred Best Books, in conducting metaphysical cock fights between Thomas Aquinas and William James. Never for a moment does it seem to occur to them that there is really very little point in reading the best, or most scientific, or most modern, or most medieval books, unless the reader is provided with a technique that permits his Self to implement in psychophysical practice the ideals set forth in these volumes.

Only two such techniques, I repeat, have ever been discovered—Alexander's and that of the mystics, Oriental and Christian. Christian mystics have tended to neglect the physical side of the total organism, with the result that they have made their supremely indirect approach to the ultimate control of all controls even more arduous than it must, in the nature of things, always be. Oriental contemplatives have not made the mistake of ignoring the body. Of the physical practices they have developed most are concerned with the direct production of certain states and symptoms; but a few seem to be aimed, though this is not specifically stated, at the mastery of the primary psychophysical control. Be that as it may, the fact remains that Alexander's technique for the conscious mastery of the primary control is now available, and that it can be combined in the most fruitful way with the technique of the mystics for transcending personality through increasing awareness of ultimate reality. It is now possible to conceive of a totally new type of education affecting the entire range of human activity, from the physiological, through the intellectual, moral, and practical, to the spiritual—an education which, by teaching them the proper use of the self, would preserve children and adults from most of the diseases and evil habits that now afflict them; an education whose training in inhibition and conscious control would provide men and women with the psychophysical means for behaving rationally and morally; an education which in its upper reaches, would make possible the experience of ultimate reality. To those who are interested in the possibilities of a new and more effective education, I heartily recommend the most enlightening of Mr Alexander's books. In *The Universal Constant in Living* they will find, along with a mass of interesting facts, the ripest wisdom of a man who, setting out 50 years ago to discover a method for restoring his lost voice, has come, by the oldest of indirect roads, to be a quite uniquely important, because uniquely practical, philosopher, educator, and physiologist.

SEVENTEEN

The *Alexander Principle and some Spiritual Disciplines*
by Fr Geoffrey Curtis, CR

(An Alexander Memorial Lecture given at the Medical
Society of London in 1972)

LADY CHAIRMAN AND all other dear Brothers and Sisters. I had
originally been asked to speak on my "experience of the Alexander
Technique and perhaps its relationship to other spiritual disciplines".
I therefore suggested the title "The Alexander Principle and other
spiritual disciplines". Some of you have scruples which I well
understand, over a title which ascribed to the Alexander Principle or
Technique a character which it has never claimed. So I altered it
readily in respect to these scruples. But clearly there is something to
be said in defence of the title originally suggested. My own experience
affirms this. The experience of everyone present will suggest or at
least excuse this conception of the Alexander Technique. For though
it does not claim to be a spiritual discipline, no one who has submitted to the education it presents has not found himself *being
disciplined spiritually.* As to the fact of discipline, I love the deliciously
crisp characteristic remark of FMA, "Anyone can do what I do, IF
they will do what I did. But none of you want the *discipline.*" That
discipline in FMA himself penetrated deep into the spirit. Perceptiveness, penitence, intelligence, persistence, the humble readiness
to begin again and again, the passion faithfully to conserve and
unsparingly to convey carried him, for all his faults, to a highly
spiritual level of self-modesty and vision. Alexander and his great
pupil, Bernard Shaw, were not mystics. They reached a similar
conviction as to the possibilities open to mankind through psychophysical re-education. They had a similar vision of the future and
kindred faith in certain biological currents of light and life which
would co-operate with mankind if they would seek steadfastly
enough to realize that vision.

But more unquestionable is the spiritual effect of the technique
on each individual learner. You will allow me to read a para-
graph from Anthony's Diary in Aldous Huxley's novel *Eyeless in
Gaza.*

At today's lesson with Miller [Miller is Alexander heavily disguised] I found myself suddenly a step forward in my grasp of the theory and practice of the technique. To learn proper use one must first inhibit all improper uses of the self. Refuse to be hurried into gaining ends by the equivalent (in personal psychophysiological terms) of violent revolution: inhibit this tendency, concentrate on the means whereby the end is to be achieved; then act. . . . Acquire the habit of inhibiting muscular bad use and you acquire thereby the art of inhibiting more complicated trains of behaviour. Not only this, there is prevention as well as cure. Given a proper correlation, many occasions for behaving undesirably just don't arise. There is an end for example of neurotic anxieties and depressions—whatever the previous history. For note: most infantile and adolescent histories are *disastrous* but only some individuals develop serious neurosis. Those precisely in whom *use of the self* is particularly bad. They succumb because resistance is poor. In practice neurosis is always associated with some kind of wrong use. (Note the typically bad physical posture of neurotics and lunatics. The stooping back, the muscular tension, the sunken head.) Re-educate, give back correct physical use. You remove a keystone of the arch constituting the neurotic personality. The neurotic personality collapses, and in its place is built up a personality in which all the habits of physical use are correct. . . . The power to cure bad behaviour seems essentially similar to the power to cure bad co-ordination. One learns this last, when learning the proper use of the self. . . . It becomes easier to inhibit undesirable impulses. Easier to follow as well as see and approve the better. Easier to put good intentions into practice and be patient, good tempered, kind, unrapacious, chaste.

I am aware that the fictional portrait of Alexander which has come down to us in the figure of Miller is amalgamated with a good deal which Huxley admired in Alexander's pet aversion, Gerald Heard. But this passage describing the Alexander Principle as a technique of education surely rings true. We have all been alive to the fact that this process of education has proved spiritually as well as physically and intellectually a powerful force of a disciplinary kind. It is true that to a certain kind of so-called spiritual discipline Alexander was strongly averse. One can understand his dislike of any association of his work with occultism, hypnosis, auto-suggestion or esotericism. These have no right to be considered as *spiritual* and seldom in the long run bear fruit in disciplined character. He might have been less

intolerant with regard to Yoga, though that little word is used to
cover several exceedingly different schemes of training and at least
two different attitudes to life. I was very glad to know of the conference held for teachers of Yoga and teachers of the Alexander
Technique; and delighted that exponents of each discipline seem to
have learnt things of value from one another, quite apart from finding
much in common. But with regard to the suggestion of a religious
thinker like Archbishop William Temple that the technique held
within itself the principle of the creativity of faith, and that of
philosophers like John Dewey and Aldous Huxley that Alexander's
discoveries had provided means by which things known theoretically
may be changed into vital experience, for these he had real sympathy.

I want to express this evening my strong conviction that both
these judgements, first with regard to Alexander's affinity with the
religious approach and secondly with regard to the benefit done to
philosophy, are true and I would like to develop them in the light of
my own experience. May I quote again from Aldous Huxley a fine
passage from the *Saturday Review of Literature* quoted in the
Alexander Journal, a simple passage which gives fine expression to
both these convictions. He is speaking, for himself, of the great flaw
in education and in the mentality of western man as a whole, the
separation and disassociation of mind and body, which Professor
Dewey also has deplored as "incarnated in religion, morals and
business as well as in science and philosophy". Huxley speaks of
Alexander as having discovered the needed educational bridge
between idealistic theory and actual practice. Books, however
enlightened, are by themselves of no avail "unless the reader is
provided with *a technique that permits his self to implement in psychophysical practice the ideals set forth in them*". He goes on:

Only two such techniques have ever been discovered—Alexander's
and that of the mystics, Oriental and Christian. Christian mystics
have tended to neglect the *physical* side of the total organism, with
the result that they have made their supremely indirect approach
to the ultimate control of all controls even more arduous than it
must, in the nature of things, always be. Oriental contemplatives
[he means non-Christian] have not made the mistake of ignoring
the body. Of the physical practices they have developed most are
concerned with the direct production of certain states and symptoms: but a few seem to be aimed, though this is not specifically
stated, at the mastery of the primary psychophysical control. Be
that as it may, the fact remains that Alexander's technique for the

conscious mastery of the primary control is now available, and that it can be combined in the most fruitful way with the technique of the mystics for transcending personality through increasing awareness of ultimate reality. It is now possible to conceive of a totally new type of education affecting the entire range of human activity, from the physiological through the intellectual, moral and practical to the spiritual—an education which by teaching them the proper use of the self would preserve children and adults from most of the diseases and evil habits that now afflict them; an education whose training in inhibition and conscious control would provide men and women with psychophysical means for behaving rationally and morally; and an education which in its upper reaches would make possible the experience of ultimate reality.

To those who are interested in the possibilities of a new and more effective education of this kind, I heartily recommend the most enlightening of Mr Alexander's books. In *The Universal Constant in Living* they will find, along with a mass of interesting facts, the ripest wisdom of a man who, setting out 50 years ago to discover a method for restoring his voice, has come, by the oldest of indirect roads, to be a quite uniquely important, because uniquely practical, philosopher, educator and physiologist.

So the Alexander Principle and Technique is to be used together with the principles and methods found in the tradition of contemplation, Christian and Oriental, to form this *new education* which is to fulfil "those highest moral and religious ideals" of which Huxley holds we have a "direct intuition". It is the Alexander Principle perhaps which will be chiefly operative in the early and basic levels: the education which in its upper reaches is to make possible the experience of ultimate reality, will be the level on which the mystical tradition is more evident. But they will both be operative together throughout.

I'm sure that many of you have a strong desire to "declare impediments" before I propose this marriage. I can quite see that the announcement of the banns even must be put off indefinitely until you can be sure that the neutrality and scientific integrity of the Alexander system of education would be preserved in such a match. But I should like to put forward a few points in favour of Huxley's prophetic vision.

First I agree with him that Christianity, the religion I know best, would gain tremendously by the general use of the Alexander Technique. This in three ways.

First, Christianity, especially western Christianity, has suffered terribly from the divorce of which both Dewey and Huxley speak between body and spirit. This ought clearly to have been impossible in the religion which is characterized as faith in the Incarnation. It would have been impossible if the Hebrew mentality in which that faith was bred had controlled its formulation throughout the early centuries. It is marvellous indeed how far it did prevail. The belief of the Manicheans that God who is spirit, as Jesus had said, cannot have created the material world, was condemned outright as heresy. The Sacraments, which show spirit as operating through material elements and making of material objects its effective symbols, are direct indications that matter belongs to God, has been redeemed and may be sanctified by Him. Nevertheless the mentality of the Greco-Roman world triumphed, at least in the west. If there is one single man who, more than any other, bears the responsibility for this, it is an African who had been a Manichean and, after conversion, found Platonic thought which sets no value on the material, the instrument through which his colossal genius might best expound his Christian faith. The name of that man was Augustine of Hippo, who still bestrides the narrow world of academic theology like a Colossus. He is the enemy of all true Kinaesthesia, a direct ancestor of Descartian man, the "ghost in the machine". A thousand, thousand text books in seminaries and conventual houses throughout the world contain passages which imply that the fleshly body is more wicked than the mind or spirit. But this is, for the Christian, falsehood and nonsense. All material things have their origin in God. The world as He made it is very good. Matter fulfils its true purpose when it is subject to spirit and a means to the self-realization of spirit. If a man is not spiritual in and through the body, he cannot be spiritual at all. The acceptance of the Alexander Technique as a cornerstone of Christian education would cure us of legacies of Platonism and of the Puritanism that is its uglier step-daughter. We should grow in the sense of the light-giving wisdom of the sacramental principle.

So the catholic instinct claims the Alexander Technique as its ally. But so with equal humility, I think, does the evangelical in its insistence on the primary need of *faith*—the necessity of "Treading our wilful doings down," of not behaving as if our life was one long procession tray-in-hand, at a serve-yourself counter. William Temple was right in marvelling at the wholesome sense of the creativity of faith in the Alexander system. You are to give your orders and not do anything to implement them. Leave that to what, to whom?—to the unknown Origin. This phrase I find in Alexander to be most crucial.

Origin has a capital O. FMA was penetrated from head to toe with the sense that man is *made in the image of God* and must leave the reconstitution of the undistorted image to this great Origin. The learning of the Alexander Technique would instil in Christians a sense of our *need of grace*. Someone might say, but Alexander relied on *nature* not on *grace*. Thank God the conceptual cleavage between nature and supernature, nature and grace which has done so much harm in western theology, is gradually seen to be at best a misleading half-truth. *Grace is everywhere*.

Thirdly, all religious folk, perhaps none more so than Christians, can benefit by learning through the Alexander Technique to avoid *end-gaining* and to pay careful attention to the *means-whereby*. These were simple terms coined by a genius, brilliantly used by Alexander with the aim of bringing home his message. Aldous Huxley erected them into a philosophy, but the philosophy needs modification. He saw that there is usually a certain affiliation between ends and means. The principle attributed to the Jesuits "The end justifies the means" is a fallacy, for the end always savours of or is characterized by the means used to gain it. A so-called peace-settlement won by violent means will be characterized by double-edged ambiguity. If I rush indecently through my business and packing, so as to get two days' rest, the rest will do less to refresh me: it will have the kind of effect produced, in the culinary world, by a half-poached, half-scrambled egg. There was genius in Alexander's conception which, as so many of his conceptions do, holds the wealth of countless life-giving analogies. As a Christian, I hold that there is a single final all-comprehensive End which is total universal love, which will cure us of all lesser end-gaining tendencies and by itself ensure the constant attention to means-whereby. But the Alexander Technique will be invaluable as a means for instilling the kind of discrimination which will ensure the living, moment to moment, of the eschatological life. A life with a view to the end and touched by the character of that end.

The Alexander Technique will make us more aware of the symbolism of the body. This was not a notion explicitly prized by Alexander. But the whole technique is implicitly impregnated with a sense of this symbolism. It could not be otherwise, as we owe it to an accomplished interpreter of Shakespeare who on the stage used physical gesture and deportment in the interests of his dramatic interpretation. Dr Grahame Fagge's lecture on the "Deeper Significance of Posture and Movement" in the *Alexander Journal* is truly Alexandrine in its character, in its boldness, its creativity, even if one would like to modify or develop considerably some of its concluding

reflections. I myself dare to hope that the teachers of the Alexander
Technique will accept explicitly this principle of the symbolism of
the body. If they do so, they will find themselves in full harmony
with the exponents of the contemplative tradition.

The extraordinary importance of Alexander's discovery with
regard to the effects of a right relationship between head, neck and
spine on the whole human organism is itself reflected in the mystical
tradition by its unbroken insistence on the spiritual importance of
uprightness. This has been best in the east, the Christian east and
the non-Christian east. It is only the western mystics who largely
neglected the importance of posture. It is true that western theologians went sadly wrong in mocking the hesychasts of Mount Athos
and their great defender, St Gregory Palamas, for their insistence
that physical deportment is a factor of salient importance in the
cultivation of the spiritual life. On the promontory of Mount Athos,
the home of 20 monasteries of the eastern Orthodox churches, there
has always been a deep conviction and a living experience of this
truth. It made me happy, when I went there to pay homage to the
monastic republic on its thousandth birthday, to find how much there
was there which implemented spiritually and psychologically the
Alexander method of education. As there were so many Russians
there in his time, it is conceivable that Tolstoy, who, though an
enemy of the church, loved the monks, may have been indebted to
a monastic source for that observation I culled from his letters: "For
me the back is an important part of the physiognomy, and especially
the place where the neck joins the back: no other part of the body so
clearly reveals lack of self-confidence and false sentiment."

The eastern Orthodox mystical tradition and that of non-Christian
orthodox mystics does far more justice to the symbolism of the body
as a whole. The centrality and vital significance of the heart has
comparatively little attention paid to it in the Alexander system. The
prayer of the heart is essential in eastern orthodox spirituality.
Considering that Jesus died of a broken heart, as is proved medically
by the two-fold flux of water and blood when his side was pierced
after death, it is not surprising that the heart of man should seem to
the faithful a locus of communion with the Eternal. There are
wonderful passages in the mystics describing the exchange of their
hearts for that of their perfect lover, Jesus. But so immense was the
tyranny of non-Christian philosophy in the west in the Roman
Catholic church that it needed the so-called "revelations of the
Sacred Heart" to St Margaret Mary Alacoque to make the west
alive again to the vital importance of this symbol. At the same time

there was a break-through in England towards a warmer, more realistic devotion, but in Protestant circles, so that the first book on the heart of Jesus was written not by a priest of the Roman church but by one of Oliver Cromwell's Protestant divines, Thomas Goodwin. The truth is that the rich vein of warm scriptural mystical devotion to the Lord Jesus flourished in Protestant England at the same time as it began anew in France. That flame has never gone out in either land. It is the reason why Roman Catholics are finding themselves so much closer to Methodists and other Protestants than Anglicans find themselves to either group.

But one tendency prevalent in classical times in the psychophysical spirituality of Mount Athos puzzled and troubled me. It seemed to smudge the record of St Gregory Palamas, the great theologian of the east, in that he defended it. This was the great emphasis laid by the monks on being conscious of the navel and the region below it as of central importance in the spiritual life of man. This I couldn't take. But I was to discern, as I will tell you, that I was wholly wrong.

Meanwhile compared with this I found Hindu and Buddhist spirituality much more congenial, especially perhaps Zen Buddhism. These supply so much that is profoundly Christian, the actualization of which has been so rare in Christianity. I mean the sense that Eternal Life is here and now available through the Sacrament of the Present Moment. It elicits a great sense of urgency. In this direction the Alexander Technique provides an analogy and a stimulus. "Here now quick always." Many splendid people have found their way back to Christianity through recourse to the oriental sources of ancient wisdom. I think of Douglas Harding, an architect who was musing in the foothills of the Himalayas on the strange fact of the holiness of India, land of such misery and corruption, when he was given an experience of enlightenment that has been fruitful in many lives—an experience which he at first found it easier to interpret in the setting of Zen Buddhism. Or I recall Lanza del Vasto, the greatest mind perhaps that I know, who lost his Christian faith in Italian universities and recovered it in India where Gandhi named him Shantidas, Servant of Peace. Such men become much in debt to Yoga, not to the secularized Yoga which flourishes so well in this city, but to that which is intent through the training of body and mind together upon an ever growing experience of the eternal beauty. This means that through a kind of transcendental meditation they find themselves as conscious as any pupil of Alexander of the essential function of the body/mind relationship in human well-being. With regard to the relation between oriental contemplation, non-Christian sources and

F

Christian contemplation, I hope you have been reading Thomas Merton's *Asian Journal*, his account of his last journey to Asia. He there says he found many contemplatives with greater assurance and serenity than he observed in his own and other Christian lands.

One grows to understand this when one hears of the pilgrimage of such Christian men and when one has met adherents of these religions. I once had the great experience of being five weeks in a Buddhist hospital with monks around. One realizes how much we have in common and how much light we can take from others to clarify and illuminate our own traditions. I humbly suggest that the Alexander Technique has much to learn even in its own field of organic reintegration and improved kinaesthesia from other disciplines. It has a great service to give and it is in giving that it will find most enrichment and illumination. I believe it is along the lines of the exploration of the symbolism of the body that it perhaps will learn most strikingly. I think it will learn a lesson that western gentility and pride, and a certain stupidity, prevented my learning on Mount Athos. Alexander teachers will learn it best, not from that promontory, but from the sages of Japan. For the great Original has granted the wise men and women of that country, in preparation and compensation perhaps for the hideous wrong done to them by nations of the west, nominally Christian, through the atomic bomb, the life-giving, world-conquering secret as to the vital centre of man—in Japanese, "Hara", the lower belly. (Read *Hara the Vital Centre*, by Karlfried von Dürkheim, Mandala Edition, Unwin 1977).

The question I ask myself at this point is: How far Christians have the grace of humility? If so, we shall be able to consider the challenge presented by the Hara tradition which is wholly contrary to our own (I am not speaking of the instructed Alexander élite)— "Chest out, belly in . . . a nation capable of taking this injunction as a general rule is in great danger." So said a Japanese in 1938 of a great western nation. Where do we believe to lie the sources of our own strength? What do we think of the region between the navel and the pelvis? Nothing much perhaps. Dr Grahame Fagg has written:

Take firstly the two main areas of tension in the back: they are the neck and the lumbar region and of course these are the two mobile parts of the spine, coming between the thoraco-abdominal region and the head above and the pelvis below. It seems to me that the self is situated in the chest and abdomen. Authority; society; parents; teachers; church; law; medicine; superego—reside in the head; Alexander was right in putting the neck-tensions first. Most of our troubles stem from conflict with society and parents, who see themselves as society's main agents in dealing with the toddler.

This conflict between self and society generates within us a sense of right and wrong as appreciated by the toddler, and we cast out the evil into the pelvis, that sink of iniquity that has to do with sex and lavatories.

Of course the writer is not speaking for himself, but of the common or nursery mind. But apart from procreation and the pleasure and happiness that belong to sex we do not think of that lower region as the source itself in ordinary life of human vitality. How significant is the disinclination of Christians in the west to mention the belly. For instance, St John shows our Lord on the last and great day of the feast of the Dedication standing up in the Temple to make a solemn promise for the sake of "those who believe on him". He does so in words that recall the prophecy of Isaiah: "If any man believes in me, out of the belly shall flow rivers of living water" (John 7.37f.). Whether the water is to flow from himself or from the believer or from both sources alike is not clear. But English translators have no right to translate *Koilia*, belly, as *heart*. The word "bowels" is similarly avoided by modern translators. We clearly disregard what St Paul calls "those parts of the body which we think less honourable. . . . But God has adjusted the body, giving the greater honour to the inferior part . . . that there may be no discord in the body" (1 Cor. 12.23 f.).

Japanese philosophers and spiritual guides hold that we have in the lower region the bond which unites us with the ground of being, the wellspring of all that is best in human life. Spirituality consists in realizing this.

If one divides people into ranks [said one of the great sages, Okado Toiajiro], the lowest is he who values his *head*. Those who endeavour only to amass as much knowledge as possible, grow heads that become bigger and so they topple over easily, like a pyramid upside down. They excel in imitating others, but neither originality nor inventiveness nor any great work is theirs. [I am not sure I don't belong to this class.]

Next come those of middle rank. For them the *chest* is most important. People with self-control, given to abstinence and asceticism, belong to this type. These are men with outward courage, but without real strength. Many of the so-called great men of history are in this category. Yet all this is not enough.

But those who regard the *belly* as the most important part and so have built the stronghold where the Divine can grow—these are the people of the highest rank. They have developed their minds as well as their bodies in the right way. Strength flows out of them and produces a spiritual condition of ease and equanimity. They do what seems good without violating any law. Those in the first category think that Science can rule Nature. Those in the second have apparent courage and discipline and know how to fight. Those in the third know what reality is. . . .

The Alexander Technique has made an incomparable contribution to civilization. It has surmounted the old dualistic thinking about man in terms of body and soul which is the hallmark of western thought, and it has given us the means of building a bridge over this gulf in ourselves and (with their co-operation) in others. This can only be achieved by the constant practice, at first under skilled aid such as you are giving, of the soul/body unity. I believe that this will be done with less perfection unless it bases itself on that vital centre in man. Spirituality, if it is to be fully Christian, must include the realization of this.

EIGHTEEN

Ordering
(Correspondence between Dr Wilfred Barlow and Fr Geoffrey Curtis)

I

Dear Father Curtis,

I was delighted to receive the typescript of the lecture which you gave to us at the Medical Society of London and since I suggested the original title, perhaps you won't mind if I comment on one or two of the points which you brought up. Anything I write is of course within an overall great appreciation of what you have written, but I think it would be fruitful to bring up a point which always has perplexed and still perplexes some Alexander teachers and students. I refer to the passage in which you say, "You are to give your orders and not do anything to implement them." To me, this implies a far too simple concept of what "ordering" implies and I would state my objection as follows.

There is no one simple method of giving "orders". Let us take the example of an Alexander student-teacher who has been working intensively for several hours and (occasionally) emerges at the end of such a session in what I expect you might consider a state of "grace", in which the "words" and the "flesh" are one and the whole organism is in a "directive state". Let us take the same student-teacher who has been absent for a few days with, perhaps, the impact of family troubles, much physical labour, much emotional stress, etc., and who returns to the training class in a somewhat tattered state, in spite of best efforts to maintain a state of Alexanderine direction throughout the troubled time. Such a person, who is in a very similar state to that of the average pupil who comes in for a lesson straight off the raucous streets of London, cannot immediately switch himself into the same "directive state" which was previously possible. The giving of orders when in a poor state cannot be the same either in its mode or in its effectiveness as it will be when one is in a supremely good state.

For this reason it is useful to think of "ordering" in the following way. Firstly it is useful to tell pupils that for a short period at the start of the lesson they should, as you put it, "give their orders and not do anything to implement them". I would call this "first-stage ordering". This period of directing at once begins to calm the mind, and such initial calming is not very different from the calming effect which might be achieved by meditation or prayer or some other repetitive mental disciplines. This effect is soon apparent to the pupil and in many disciplines the effect has been found to be so beneficial that it has seemed that by persevering in such a way (and without elaboration) a sufficient "state of grace" can be achieved. By inhibiting and directing, the inborn accuracy will, it is hoped, assert itself. It does however appear, unhappily, that in spite of such a discipline of inhibiting and ordering, misuses do not change sufficiently, and Huxley's goals of being "good tempered, patient, unrapacious, and chaste" are often not very obvious.

It was, however, precisely in his refusal to accept this "first-stage" effect as being sufficient that Alexander made his most meaningful contribution—to what I would call "stage two ordering". This "stage two" of ordering is one of *particularizing*, in which what was in the first stage only a broad outline of directions is now used in more detail in the essential Alexander procedure as described in Chapter 1 in his *Use of the Self*. It was here that he described his totally novel procedure of introducing a stimulus (self-selected), the response to which was to be *inhibited* and replaced by *direction* and by the choice of either (1) to respond, (2) to continue inhibiting or (3) to carry out some quite different reaction: in this way he gave himself some freedom of choice and at last began to alter his automatic misuses.

This second stage in fact provides most of the meat of an Alexander lesson and in this stage the teacher (who is the "stimulus") teaches the pupil the bodily meaning of the orders and how to put them together in relationship to his body. In this phase the pupil's attention will actually be directed on to the particular region of the body which is being worked on, although within the general framework of what we have called "the total pattern". (I am sure you will realize the descriptive difficulties here, but in this stage two, *more* rather than *less* detail is required—all of us are capable of carrying a large number of "orders", much in the way that the letters of the alphabet can become words and then the words become sentences.)

It is after working in this way for a considerable time that a third stage of ordering becomes possible—the stage of "transformation" where a quite different level of directing is suddenly "given". In this stage "you are to give your orders and not do anything to implement them" since they have now become incarnate in psychophysical wholeness—singers who have had much training in both voice and Alexander, sometimes say that in this state they only have to think what they have to sing and it appears.

Unfortunately, for many people the Alexander discipline seems to have become equated with the first stage of ordering. It has become apparent to me over nearly 40 years of Alexander that very many teachers and students find such satisfaction in this first stage that they do not easily find their way through to the third stage and may therefore tolerate in themselves degrees of misuse which make the attainment and maintenance of the third stage extremely difficult. These misuses have to be clearly perceived and dealt with by "second stage" ordering (and by all the knowledge which this stage requires).

I wonder if my three stages of "ordering" have parallels. I see that Chomsky talks of three levels—surface structure, deep structure and "transformation": and that certain mystics talk of there being three stages Purging, Knowledge (of wrong) and Unifying. Practitioners of, for example, transcendental meditation whom I have seen, appear not to have progressed beyond stage one, and their procedure seems to be a form of self-hypnosis.

The other point which I would like to take up with you is the question of the rôle of symbolism in the Alexander Technique. I would resist utterly the very simplified view which Dr Fagg and yourself seem to take, that specific regions of the body can be related to specific feelings: e.g. the chest being the seat of courage. The last 50 years have seen such symbolism exploited to the full by the Freudians and post-Freudians who, for example, might suggest that the pen with which I write is in fact a male sexual organ or, in the case of the Jungians, that a female breast is symbolized in dreams by a hill. It has become clear that a psychotherapist's patient will dream up dreams for his therapist in whatever symbolism that particular therapist may prefer—a Jungian's patient dreams Jungian dreams, and so on—and whilst someone may perhaps insist that for them the use of the chest is to be equated with courage or timidity, this (it seems to me) is only the case *once this equation has been suggested*. Symbols, on this view, are manufactured, not absolutes: courage and timidity can equally be equated with the jaw, or the shoulders or the buttocks, as actors know.

Or, to take another example, the symbol of the cross could quite fruitfully be used in an Alexander context as a symbol of the body lengthening (the upright stroke of the cross) and widening (the horizontal portion). Such a symbolism could be an inspiring reminder of human potentiality and of re-birth through the Alexander orders. "Crucifixion", in this scheme of symbolism, would come about when we "create a crooked cross" to which we habitually fix ourselves. The Alexander "cross of Good-Use" certainly involves suffering if it is to be constantly refined, but the "suffering" is spread over a lifetime each time we inhibit the crooked cross of Habit. An "anxious pause" when we inhibit is unavoidable: indeed, it is to prevent such anxiety ("suffering") that we end-gain—but I must not stray off into this fascinating topic!

Wilfred Barlow
March 1976

II

A reply from Father Geoffrey Curtis, CR
Dear Dr Barlow,
You will have already received through the secretary of your society an expression of my sincere gratitude for your kind and deeply interesting letter. I am sure you are right in charging me with the wrong kind of simplification—I believe the French word is *"simplisme"*! "You are to give your orders and not to do anything to implement them"—this is my own overall impression of the principle that the Alexander teacher seeks to convey throughout the whole course of his teaching. But no doubt there are many stages and modifications in the "ordering" directed: and a great variety of kinds of particularization. These will differ not only for each pupil with whom the teacher has to do, but from lesson to lesson with the same pupil. The foundation of the ordering seems to me to have been Alexander's conviction that the human organism has its own deep wisdom and must be trusted, to a large extent and at all stages, to recover this. Its innate grace, rooted in the fact that it is created in the image of the Origin, must be allowed its freedom: but we must trust to this and be open to it.

The analogy between the teaching of the Alexander Technique and the direction of the Christian soul has always been clear to me and has become progressively more so. The three stages which issue from conversion are, as you indicate, closely parallel to those stages with which the Alexander instructor is familiar. Purgation, illumination and union are traditional categories. But all these issue from the vital light-giving experience of conversion which comprehends by anticipation all three. So there is a real danger that the convert, after his first life-giving experience of new insight into reality, and of his own already actual potentiality of transformation—the experience the

Orientals call *Samsara*—will find such satisfaction in this that he won't advance any further along the hard road towards union. But there is much in the way of learning and inhibiting and trusting which is needed before the content of that first experience can be truly appropriated.

But in both schemes—that of kinaesthesia and that of spiritual perception and training—isn't the main refrain "inhibit your own misuses, mistrust your own efforts, trust the organism and its own intrinsic grace"? I can well see that it is only in the first stage and in the last that the principle as I put it can be stated without much safeguarding and modification and particularization. But the accent throughout is surely on the *givenness* of grace. In fact all the effort, watchfulness, docility and patience inculcated are directed, aren't they? to the inhibition of one's own efforts and the mistrusting of what to oneself seems right: to the careful avoidance of setting your mind, as self-centred man always does, on the ends desired with disregard for the means taken to secure the ends, ends which will certainly be qualified by the means employed. The whole conflict between the Augustinian doctrine of the primacy, in fact the irresistibility of Grace, and the teaching of Pelagius, our countryman—that human effort is necessary in the quest of salvation—this conflict seems to me to be closely parallel to the struggle in which the teacher of the Alexander Technique must engage in order that misuse may be inhibited and that one item after another of daily bodily procedure may be allowed or trusted by his pupil to find fulfilment in the natural way, a way that seems almost suggested by the human organism itself. We must not trust our own efforts to secure the ends we desire. It is to inhibiting such ingrained inclinations that our efforts must henceforth be largely given. But there must also be much watchfulness with openness to co-operate with the intrinsic grace and wisdom of the organism. I hope I haven't got this all wrong.

As regards the rôle of symbolism in teaching the Alexander Technique, I have no doubt that I over-simplified. I am of course aware that there is a vast variety of codes of such symbolism of the bodily organs, differing from one culture to another and from this psychotherapist to the next. But despite these differences there is a general conviction that the body and its organs do represent and express certain operations of the human spirit of which the body is the sacrament. Moreover, these different codes do have a good deal of common ground. In the four cultures that I know best, Greek, Latin, Hebrew and Anglo-Saxon, despite much difference of emphasis and some surprising contrasts, there is far more unity than difference. If you add to these the Chakras of Oriental physiology, there is further corroboration of this common intuition (or congeries of intuition).

Yes, in the scheme of Alexander also "the crooked cross" of self-centred indulgence becomes the Holy cross of death-to-self which becomes the victorious cross—the instrument and sign of the triumph of love, but not without suffering. Thank you for pointing out the fruitfulness of this symbol.

You are of course right too about the need of detailed direction—particularizing. The spiritual counsellor has to deal analogously with a second stage which requires particular monitions with a view to helping the learner to get rid of apparently almost congenital habits of misuse. But he feels all the time that the chief value of these monitions is that it allows the learner to feel that he is doing something himself towards the attainment of wholeness (salvation). This is *partly* at least a concession to his all but incurable egoism. This stage includes what is called "acquired contemplation". The three stages, as I mentioned, are usually called the purgative, the illuminative and the unitive lives. Acquired contemplation comes towards the close of the illuminative phase. Its acquisition is certainly aided by the directions given to cure particular failings and to promote wholesome instincts and habits—these are not merely a sop to activism! But I hope you would agree that the innate wisdom of the "Origin"—the spirit-quickened wisdom of the image of God within the redeemed—is the primary factor in the liberation of the learner. This enables him to receive the "sudden gift" of that "quite different level" of living of which you write. This "transformation" in which the "orders" are found to "have become incarnate in psychophysical wholeness", is analogous to the unitive stage of the Christian spiritual life, a stage often characterized by "infused contemplation": a stage when the Pauline principle "Christ in you, the hope of glory" becomes a living experience. "I have been crucified with Christ, and yet I live; yet not I, for the life I live is mine through the faith of our Lord Jesus Christ who loved me and gave himself for me." The analogies between these two wholly *distinct*, but not wholly *separable* kinds of development are, as you have implied, very close.

Yours sincerely,

Geoffrey Curtis
13.10.1976

APPLICATIONS

ARTISTIC

NINETEEN

Alexander's Ideas and Visual Art
by Dr Wilfred Barlow

ARTHUR WALEY WROTE of a certain Chinese painter that when drunk used to dip his head in a pail of ink and flop it on to the painting silk. Marvellous mountains, lakes and trees appeared by magic: this is perhaps best seen as a case of painting with an unusually large brush, requiring an unusually free neck, but it is not an important application of Alexander's technique to art! The fact is that if one wants to know what a knowledge of Alexander's training (and the ideas it implies) can do for the artist—and that means, to take the question in its most interesting sense, how it will affect his work—the answer is unfortunately, that very few facts so far exist. Nor will any clear generalizations be possibly until a large number of artists have been through the experience which the Alexander training entails. Clearly the better the artist, the more developed their artistic personalities, the more important their evidence will be. We have the opinions in Chapter 20 of one painter, George Bruce, and these are interesting opinions since he is not only Secretary of the Royal Society of Portrait Painters, but he is also a trained Alexander teacher. Apart from this, very little has been written by artists so far, and all one can do is speculate on possible effects, taking what is known about the way the creative instincts of artists seem to work as one's basis.

The value to the artist of information about the facts of body-use is limited. At the anatomical level, it produced, for example, the by no means negligible illustrations attributed to Vesalius. They are not by any means what we understand nowadays by anatomical illustrations, for they were the product of an age when intellectual curiosity could embrace several abilities. They were made at a time—the first time for centuries—when the words became real to man: "Thine is the earth and the fullness thereof": and the grandeur and vitality of these anatomical figures, making typical renaissance gestures, might perhaps remind us—in the way that the illustrations in *Gray's Anatomy* do not—that the Alexander training implies a renaissance and unfolding of the whole personality.

Indeed, for the creative artist whose work is based on observation, the Alexander training is bound to open up a whole world of nuances, from the smallest gestures to movements of the whole body—or rather give them for him the infinitely greater significance which comes from understanding. What will be most interesting, however, when it becomes possible to trace it, will be the effect of Alexander training on the deeper mental levels, expressed in images often unconsciously chosen. A well-known sculptor, who came to me for lessons, shortly afterwards put on an exhibition at the Hanover Galleries. All of the works which he showed, except one, were done before he had had lessons. The critic of the *New Statesman*, who knew nothing about his Alexander lessons, wrote the following review of his exhibition: "Mr X's new sculptures are concerned with the human figure. All but one of them are unsatisfactory for a reason which has both formal and human implications: the force and intention of the movements remain *exterior* to each figure, they never grow from within it. The arms stand out like disturbed pendulums, but the bodies themselves are dead weights, lacking vitality. In the one exception" [and this is the reason for quoting this review] "the upward thrust seems to be determined by the whole body." This one exception was the work which was done *after* the sculptor had started his Alexander lessons and might reasonably be attributed to the lessons which he had had. When many more good artists have taken this training, it will be fascinating to see its effects on the presentation of images and ideas which crop up throughout the artists' life.

All this is in the future. But if there is very little to be said for now about artists, there is a good deal more if one approaches the subject from the other way round and considers the actual works of art themselves, and what a knowledge of the Alexander training can do for art appreciation.

Here one is on much more solid ground.

Douglas Newton has suggested to me that one might start by taking as an example the bronze heads from Ife in Nigeria, since not much is known about them and they can be considered on their own merit. In lesser works these heads would be said to have assurance; but such is their forceful simplicity that they can be truly called grand. Assurance is allied to poise: and that is part of the secret of these heads. Their effect is produced to some extent by the balance of the head upon the neck.

These heads are obviously portraits, and their head-neck balance has been drawn from life, rather than from an idealized pre-set as in Egyptian art. (The fallacy dies very hard that all Egyptian art was formalized and ossified throughout the long period of its existence; and that that might be taken as accounting for what is considered the rigidity of its figures.) But applying Alexander's ideas, one can see that though the *form* of the body (particularly of the limbs) was stylized, the *positions* of the head, neck and trunk were not necessarily so—they are a consequence of the way the body is held rather than a piece of artistic geometry.

The Ife heads have been compared by some to Greek art: they have even been attributed to Greek influences. If we consider specifically *what* Greek art, we find that they most resemble the archaic sculpture. In the heads of figures from Olympia one finds the same subtle degree of formalization, the same nobility, and the same perfect tenure of the head and neck. I should suggest that this directly contributes to those qualities which make us, almost instinctively, today prefer archaic Greek art to the later Greco-Roman art which first excited the artists who rediscovered it. By the third century, a flaccidity had crept into the whole head-neck-body relationship: and compared with the Apollo from Olympia, the Belvedere Apollo seems unpleasantly lax in pose.

Writing about Piero della Francesca, Sir Kenneth Clark made the important observation that he has risen to his present great position over the last 50 years or so—the period that has also seen the revolution in our taste for Greek art and in our increased appreciation of Alexander body-use. He comments, "strangely enough they [Piero's paintings] remind us . . . of [Greek] works which Piero can never have seen, as we know it from the sculpture of Olympia. . . ." But if we look at them side by side is it not true that this effect, partly at least, derives from the head-neck relationship as Piero painted it, and as the Greeks carved it? The importance of this element in Piero's painting is emphasized by Sir Kenneth Clark when he writes about the "Madonna of the Misericordia": "The head is in no way a mask . . . this is largely due to the superb column of the neck, where, for the first time, we see one of the basic elements of his art."

The same question arises as in Egyptian art: To what extent are any of these figures idealizations and to what extent based on reality? The answer may be that Piero della Francesca and the archaic Greek sculptors had all seen types of the people they carved or painted. Probably the whole race was nearer this ideal in archaic Greece, judging by figures in minor works which inclined to realism. It may not be true that a general change of physique had taken place by a few centuries later but a change in the ideals certainly had—the Belvedere Apollo had become an idealized version.

"Good-use", as described by Alexander, seems in this sense to have been used by artists as an expressive formula. Its opposite extreme has also been used, for example, by such a painter as Grünevald. In his Isenheim altar-piece, the utmost dramatic force is wrung out of the figures by their wry attitudes and the distorted placing of their heads in relation to their bodies. To an equal degree, Alexandrian good-use has been used to express the no less great extremes of serenity. Its presence seems to be one of the hallmarks of the classical artist, its absence a sign of the romantic artist.

It is interesting to consider the work of Picasso, who, for most of his life, has been a romantic artist (sometimes to the point of being a sentimental one) although there can be seen a constant harking back to classicism. His early paintings during the Blue and Pink periods of 1902–1906 show the heads of his harlequins and paupers drooping not only down in front but with an inclination to one side, sometimes almost at right-angles to the spine. This attitude occurs even in his self-portraits: with its rather sugary pathos it must have been part and parcel of his whole view of life at the time, and it is to be found in many pictures of the Negro and Cubist period which followed, for all their apparent austerity. But in his first classic period in 1920, we find the heads consistently as the Greeks saw them. These two trends in his work subsequently constituted a balance of power which may give a clue to the way in which his most surprising versions of the human form may be read.

These ideas are obviously limited in their application, and although I have heard many Alexandrians express distaste for paintings which depict misuse, a knowledge of Alexander could never be used as a criterion of artistic value. I suspect though, that as far as the human form is concerned, most Alexandrians would, over the long term, feel more at home with the classic than the romantic mood.

One should not perhaps close this brief consideration of the visual arts without mentioning a point which is often made—that the Alexander teacher is himself engaged in an artistic activity when he is working on the human form to re-educate it. A recent definition of a sculptor describes him as someone who is manipulating, modifying and re-ordering his material, and on this definition the Alexander teacher might be perhaps considered to be a human sculptor. Indeed I have myself been invited to give a lecture at one of the art colleges on "working with flesh"! The fact remains that it is an aesthetically most satisfying spectacle to watch a well-used Alexander teacher gradually coaxing his subject into a form which is more alive and co-ordinated.

TWENTY

A Painter's Training
by George J. D. Bruce

MUCH CONTEMPORARY ART and abstract painting is with little if any order, results being largely empirical, often relying on mostly *accidental* happenings, such as in Tachism. Such accidental happenings have no place in art which is in the great classical tradition. An artist working in this tradition, which has continued for nearly 1,000 years up to the mid-twentieth century, had to have a basic training in drawing, design, tone and colour relationships. Accidental happenings had no place in his work.

The neglect of such basic training, a neglect which began to take place widely from about the Impressionists onwards, has had a marked effect on contemporary painting, much of which can hardly come under the heading of "art" at all. Indeed a sound teaching in these basics has become almost unavailable today, as the older artists die, leaving many of the rising generations of art teachers largely untrained in these fundamental principles. Without such training, it is impossible for work to be carried out on a truly rational basis, with a systematic step-by-step build-up. With such a training, however, the artist is not going to be side-tracked from his original intended objective and if a painting runs into difficulties during its development, his basic training will indicate that the difficulties can usually be put down to a weakness of drawing, tone, colour, design or texture.

It is precisely when such difficulties do appear—in developing an idea from conception to completion—that the value of an Alexander-trained mind will come to the fore. With the constantly changing and developing situation taking place on the canvas, the eye of the painter who has had Alexander lessons will more easily be able to keep the whole project under dispassionate review, and he will more easily be able to observe deviations which may distract from the total forward progression of the work.

The dependence of an artist on the way in which he uses himself comes about in the following way. In simple terms, consider the type of artist whose work is based on *observation*: having seen the subject through his eyes, his brain then has to instruct the hand to manipulate his brush or pencil in such a way as to express his intention. Owing to the infinite complexity of Nature, there has always to be a great simplification in such expression. The skill with which he expresses himself cannot only be manual, the result of training and craftmanship, but it must be mental also in that his brain is sifting and selecting the available material. Such sifting and selection must inevitably be affected by his state of mind, which, of course, is where an Alexander-trained painter must stand to gain immensely.

To take one example, the first mentioned of the five headings which are essential to a trained artist, *Drawing* is not the ability to make straight lines or perfect circles freehand but an expression on a flat surface, of forms and their relative axes, actions and interactions with one another in three dimensional space. In talking of such actions of forms in space, we have a definite affinity between "drawing" and the Alexander concept of "ordering" or "directing". Both are concerned with relative axes, actions and interactions and positions of the whole sum of the human form. The Alexander orders are concerned with the relativity in space of a part or parts of the structure of the body, one to another, and the direction for these to take up (e.g. lengthening and widening the back).

To summarize, an Alexander training will affect the artist's work (i) from a point of view of intelligent selection of the material available, (ii) in better use of himself when handling his tools and materials whilst expressing those selections, and (iii) in the ability to retain a detached total control over the often rapidly changing situation which is taking place as the work progresses.

Lastly, and by no means least, a continual application of Alexander's principle, producing a clarity of mind uncluttered by irrelevancies and minutiae will surely further the development of the painter's intellect, thereby having a profound effect on the strength and directness of his work. It will also promote the greatest possible development of his own individual personality and perception of the world around him.

TWENTY-ONE

Musicians and the Technique
by Hugo Cole

ANY MUSICIAN WHO has practised the Alexander Technique is likely to feel a special interest in teaching books of past and present; in accounts of past performers; and in the platform behaviour of today's performers. He will wonder how far teachers and performers of past centuries were aware of the significance of visibly small posture variations, or of anything we would describe as *manner of use*. He would like to know what aspects of Alexander teaching were foreshadowed or paralleled by others; and how many of those who today analyse performing techniques or philosophize about the art of performance are, consciously or unconsciously, indebted to Alexander. Watching live performers, he may know of some who have practised the technique, and will observe which bring it with them on to the concert platform. Of the others, many seem to be in urgent need of the technique; but there are also those who appear to get along without it very well. Would they all in fact benefit from the technique? And just what is it that the technique has to offer musicians that is not available from other sources?

From the Past to the Present
No dark age is ever quite so dark as it looks to those who live later, in times of relative enlightenment. Because nothing is said in most eighteenth- and nineteenth-century teaching books about posture, internal muscular states, weight-distribution, tension or balance of moving parts, we should not assume that there was no awareness of such matters. Important directives were sometimes deliberately omitted because a teacher wanted to keep his secrets to himself (as in Chinese lute-notation books which omit the last chapter). More often, the books were only intended to be teaching aids, providing *material for practice*. It was understood that the use of the material was to be decided by the teacher, and that demonstration and manipulation could be effective where words were inadequate—a view which Alexander teachers might share. Emphasis is generally laid on the solution of mechanical problems. Duport's valuable and detailed book on cello technique is explicitly titled *Treatise on fingering*. C. P. E. Bach, in the "Essay on the true art of playing

keyboard instruments" does indeed mention stiffness—but only to
recommend that the pupil simplifies rapid repeated-note passages
that cause it. Leopold Mozart's *Violinschule* goes into some detail in
describing good playing positions, and also emphasizes the need to
avoid stiffness. The implication seems to be that, if the right physical
position is found, other problems will sort themselves out; thus, the
pupil is told to practise standing close to a wall so that his right elbow
cannot rise too high.

During the nineteenth century, instrumental teachers still tended
to think in terms of mechanical solutions, taking the "commonsense"
view that the active and visible movements specific to a job are what
must be mastered at all costs. Innovators concerned themselves with
the outward mechanics of technique, and stressed the need to drill
fingers by repetition of every sort of exercise, ensuring "correct"
playing position, if necessary, by mechanical means. J. B. Logier,
who considered himself "an instrument in the hands of Providence
for changing the whole system of musical education", had a great
success with the chiroplast, a device which confined the pianist's
wrists between two horizontal brass rails, and the fingers in compart-
ments of the width of the piano keys, so that they could only move
vertically, thus ensuring "correct" playing positions.

Crude mechanical devices were still being advertised in the inter-
war years. Szigeti, in his book *Szigeti on the Violin*, describes a set of
instruments on sale in 1927, including an extensor to be opened and
shut by the fingers, while the wrist, in moving backwards and
forwards, simulates a *détaché* bowing; and a wooden roll to which an
iron dumb-bell is attached by a canvas band. The violinist, holding
the roll at shoulder height, pulls the weighted band up by rotating
the roll with fingers and thumb of the right hand. And even today,
areas of darkness persist. There are still violin teachers who advocate
the holding of a telephone book under the right upper arm to
immobilize it while practising wrist bowing.

The first English teacher to analyse movements in detail and to
consider internal states as well as external actions seems to have been
the pianist Tobias Matthay, who published his *Act of Touch* in 1902,
and summed up a lifetime's work and experience in *The Visible and
Invisible in Piano Technique* in 1932. Matthay distinguished six types
of arm-functioning, four "optional" and two "compulsory". Endless
qualifications and refinements of ideas on arm-vibration touch, forearm rotation, weight-transfer touch, illustrate the difficulty of putting
into words subtle observations of body-functioning, and the ease
with which specialists can involve themselves in minute classification

processes. He is insistent that the quality of sound, as well as the intensity, can be altered by touch-variations; a view in conflict with physicists' findings. Like other laymen, he is eager to seize on scientific findings that support his views. His distinction of two sorts of muscle: one to do the work, the other to maintain position, based on the work of the Australian Dr John Hunter in the 1920s, over-simplifies the real problems.

Yet much of what Matthay says is, from the Alexandrian point of view, of great interest:

> There is no such thing as "muscular habit"; there is only "mental habit" . . .
> You must be able to recall the sensation accompanying the correct exertion or movement of the limb, and to acquire such sensations of right doing, you must *experiment* . . .
> [On invisible changes of state] The trouble all along has been, that since these *exertions* are not disclosed by movements, they completely escaped notice; and teachers of the past, unaware of these facts, were unable to help their pupils . . .
> You can only achieve free action of the limb by *wishing* it to be free.

On general posture, he is not very explicit:

> DO NOT SIT LIKE A HUNCHBACK. It is distinctly unhealthful, and of no profit technically . . . Freely and easily keep your body erect, or nearly so. A slight leaning forward from the hips is more comfortable for some. Playing freely, with the constantly recurring relaxations of your upper arm and shoulder, is likely to tempt you to relax also the muscles that keep your body erect. Have a care that this does not happen.

Matthay went a good way in relating movement and internal muscular states of upper arm, forearm, and head, one to another. He suggested the inevitable involvement of the organism-as-a-whole when he wrote: "Should you play stiffly and badly, you are almost compelled to sit stiffly and more or less immobile." If he had accepted the converse of this proposition: that if you sit stiffly you will also play stiffly; he would have got near to Alexander's basic belief. It seems probable that Matthay had heard of Alexander's work. He refers disparagingly to "a world-reeling Discovery, viz., the teaching

of Technique by means of 'CONSCIOUS-Mental-Muscular-Control' ";
a discovery he claims to have anticipated 30 years before in *The Act
of Touch.*

Another pianist and teacher of the inter-war years came still
closer to Alexander's thinking in her views on inhibition and
body-awareness. Lilias Mackinnon stressed the need to inhibit
unthoughtout actions and to prepare every movement in advance. In
sight-reading, she insisted that it was possible, by reading the music
through and *thinking* the performance in advance, to prepare so well
that you need never make a mistake. In practice, you must rehearse
only right actions. She described a process of "progressive relaxation" in which you attended to each part of the body in turn, saying
to yourself: "my left arm is relaxed ... my left hand is relaxed ...",
the form of the phrase encouraging you to observe rather than to take
action. In her book *Music by Heart*, she refers to Coué's "Law of
reversed effort": "the harder he tries, the less he is able" and adds:
"the necessity for non-interference by the conscious mind is demonstrated in the case of all actions that have become habitual through
repetition ... it cannot be repeated too often that the rôle of the
musician's intelligence lies in selecting and educating the habits, in
correcting them if need be". And, later: "Freedom is a better word
[than relaxation] for the desired muscular condition, which helps to
bring about the right mental state 'attention minus effort'; when
mind and body are free from strain, then habits perform with
proficiency." This seems to be in line with Alexander's ideas. But
on posture, she can do no better than quote a friend, Miss G. Routh,
who advises: "Pianists should sit up with arched back, without
relaxing at the waist." As she refers to others who have influenced
her, but not to Alexander, I imagine that she had not come across
his work.

Scientific or semi-scientific research into external mechanical
problems or into the physiology of instrumental playing has not yet
proved to be of much use to practising musicians. Thus, Percival
Hodgson's *Motion Study in Violin Playing* analysed bowing-
movement patterns by means of cyclographs: light-tracings of
bow-heel and elbow movements. That these provide new information
is not to be questioned; but it is hard to see how they can be employed
to improve use or technique. James Ching, a pianist with specialized
knowledge of physiology, wrote several books on piano technique
emphasizing the importance of tension- and relaxation-states within
the joints, and describing playing-positions in some detail. These
books, however useful as "teaching-aids", do not take us much

further towards an understanding of basic problems of mental-physical co-ordination. More recent books on violin technique have shown considerable interest in what the Alexander teacher would describe as *good-use.* Herbert Whone, in *The Simplicity of Playing the Violin,* begins with two chapters on "Feeling awareness in the body" and "Stance and balance". He speaks of the body which is "more often than not blind to itself" and of the need to cultivate "feeling-awareness" and a state of minimal tension (in the bowing arm) to which the player can return at will. Kato Havás in *A New Approach to Violin Playing* describes the "condition of looseness" throughout the body that allows the player freedom. She writes: "A state of relaxation must not be looked on as something vague and negative. It ought to become just as definite a feeling as the feeling of cramp. On the other hand it is not enough to say 'relax', 'loosen up'. Such a direction becomes of real value only when every step towards achieving relaxation and looseness has been so clearly explained and experienced that it would seem ridiculous to do anything else." She realizes as clearly as an Alexander teacher the importance of cross-connections and cross-influences in tension patterns; that a poor spiccato (bouncing bow) may be caused by an uncertain left (fingering) hand, and that bowing insecurities may lead to tensions and malfunctioning in the fingering hand.

In both Whone and Havás, we catch undoubted echoes of Alexander's teaching; which is hardly surprising when the technique is taught at several major musical institutions and when so many young string players have first-hand knowledge of its application. But there are no connections, hidden or explicit, between Alexander and the Japanese violin teacher Suzuki. Suzuki's fame rests mainly on his success with very small children. There are several points of resemblance between his methods and aims and those of the Alexander teacher:

1 The importance of good posture is emphasized from the very beginning. Before children handle their violins at all, simple movements are practised (without instruments) rather as the basic actions of standing, sitting, and so on are rehearsed "out of context" by Alexander pupils.

2 Suzuki is concerned with the whole individual. Children come to him to learn the violin; but he has been known to say to ambitious parents: "He will become a noble person through his violin playing—isn't that enough?" Alexander teachers do not talk much about "nobility"; but they do emphasize the connection between all forms of mental and physical activity. As Alexander said: "Talk

about a man's individuality and character—it's the way he uses himself."

3 Suzuki insists on the possibility of change for all. He believes, as Alexander did, that habits of good-use can be acquired by deliberate action, and that any child can acquire the physical and mental skills needed to play the violin if the clearly-ordered course he has devised for them is followed.

One of the most remarkable features of Suzuki's own teaching has been his success in "making eager" (to use his own phrase). He has been able to maintain the spirit of enthusiasm and discovery through the laborious and unspectacular early stages, implanting the most subtle skills in quite tiny children by ensuring the co-operation of their parents and by introducing game-like elements into the teaching process. Alexander teachers, who would prefer to spend less time in putting right what has gone wrong, might well study Suzuki's methods. Many Suzuki teachers have been trained and the system is widely used in America; the question of how far it is adaptable for western use, and how far Suzuki teaching—without Suzuki himself— remains the same thing, is still subject to debate.

Brass players inhabit a different world from other instrumentalists; a world with its own customs, traditions, and standards. The ancestors of today's trumpeters and hornists were soldiers and huntsmen. Anthony Baines, in his *Brass Instruments: Their History and Development*, points out that the chief function of the military trumpeter was "to inflame the army" and quotes Shakespeare's vivid evocation of trumpeting in *Troilus and Cressida*: "Thou, trumpet . . . Come, stretch thy chest and let thy eyes spout blood." Portraits of brass players show a gradual easing of tension in facial muscles over the centuries. The world of military music was, in fact, one of the only places where questions of posture and movement for musicians were treated systematically and seriously. Lieutenant Geary, of the Royal Artillery Band, even introduced a system of precise and timed movements for the raising and blowing of all band instruments, and the *correct posture* for every instrument can also be found illustrated in Henry Farmer's *History of the Royal Artillery Band*. But what posture! Nor did the leading conservatoire teachers of the nineteenth century have much to suggest. To quote Anthony Baines again:

Dauprat, author of the Parisian Horn Méthode held in highest repute (1824), could have given this matter no thought at all, merely quoting from the Conservatoire's singing tutor: "To breathe in, the belly must be flattened, swelling the chest, and to breathe out the belly returns slowly to its natural position and the chest is lowered" . . . though to be fair, Domnich mentions the diaphragm inhalation, and achievement of a "well-controlled and efficient expiration" as opposed to the "old manner of blowing with the chest".

It was the cornet players, perhaps less bound by convention than the trumpeters, who introduced, in the early years of this century, "no-pressure systems" in which tension of the lips played a main part in controlling the pitch of a note. It was also the cornettists who made the most positive moves towards diaphragm breathing: "Seventy years ago, pupils of Petit in France were made to place a hand upon the stomach to check that air is drawn in by pulling down the diaphragm not by raising the chest" (Baines). Today, "experience is preceded by accurate training; pupils are taught to produce very deliberately and positively the exact lip frequency required, learning to do this by extensive practice on the mouthpiece alone . . . or with the lips alone (lip buzzing)". This sort of rational pre-rehearsal of significant actions is in line with Alexander teaching, and suggests that during the last decades there has indeed been a general move towards thinking, rather than instinctive, approaches to technical problems.

I shall say little of singing-teaching. It would take an expert, which I am not, to compare and assess the countless methods and systems which have appeared during the last three or four centuries. Because they deal in non-visibles, singing teachers avoid the danger that threatens violin and piano teachers: that they may fill their books with minute descriptions of purely mechanical actions. Their weakness lies in the fact that they are forced to describe sounds and physical sensations in metaphors that are often almost meaningless for those who are not advancing along their own particular lines.

Elster Kay, in his book on *bel canto*, lists some of the descriptive phrases coined by teachers in their efforts to give pupils the required sensation. Pupils are told to lay all the vowels on the vocal cords and the consonants on the teeth; to think of a ladder, or two ladders, in the head, a biscuit mould and Hoover in the mouth and a chimney in the throat. The upper jaw is to be thought of as a long pointed bird's beak which, during singing, stabs into an apple. Where every teacher has his own set of images, it is hardly surprising that controversy continues to rage over the various ways of producing the voice and their relative merits.

There have, of course, been specific problems and differences of
opinion over "correct" methods of breathing. The long controversy
over high (upper-chest) breathing and low (diaphragmatic) breathing
came to a head in 1887 when Emil Behnke and Lennox Browne
published their *Voice, Speech and Song*. Before that time, singers had
often aimed at the great chest-expansions of army athletes, while
some teachers recommended "clavicular breathing"—the use of
muscles in the neighbourhood of the collarbone to raise the upper
ribs. Rubini is supposed to have broken a collarbone as a result of
using the method to deliver a high B flat. Today, it seems that most
singing teachers encourage the pupil in a manner of breathing that
involves the broadening of the base of the cone that constitutes the
thorax, with the accompanying flattening downwards of the diaphragm, that might also be suggested by Alexander teachers. On
matters of "non-doing" there is also common ground to be found
between Alexander teachers and some singing teachers. Joyce
Warrack, in her article "The indirect approach to singing", quotes
from Vincenzo Vannini's *Della Voce Umana*: "Nature's means are
essentially simple, it is only we who complicate matters with our
pretentious attempts to be helpful. . . . All that the singer can do is to
remain a spectator! He must cultivate an attitude of intelligent
laziness. . . . Nature has no need of our assistance."

Present and Future
The teaching books and methods I have mentioned seem to confirm
the belief that, over the last 60 years or so, we have come to think of
ourselves, and the ways in which we function, in rather different
terms. No longer do we necessarily regard our bodies and minds as
sealed systems, like those electrical appliances that arrive lubricated
for life, with a solemn warning that under no circumstances should
the user tamper with the mechanism. Psychologists, yoga teachers,
practical philosophers of all kinds and, of course, Alexander teachers
encourage us to believe that patterns of behaviour are not fixed
once-for-always and that we can do more than accept, fatalistically,
whatever peculiar physical and mental habits appear to be built in
to our systems. Thirty years ago, if an orchestral violinist suffered
from trembling bow during the Prelude to *Lohengrin*, or found his
arm seizing up after playing repeated semiquavers in a Liszt Tone
Poem, the chances are that he would have put it down to *nerves* or
cramp and left it at that, hoping that it would not happen again.
Eric Coates described the neuritis that plagued him when he was
leading the violas in the Queen's Hall orchestra. Today, he would

have the choice between going to a psychologist who would have told him that he was longing to leave the orchestra to devote himself to composition, or going to an Alexander teacher, who might well have eased his physical distress—and, perhaps, compelled him to recognize the existence of an underlying psychological problem.

The biggest problem comes when there is no problem. How can anyone persuade young performers, whose physical apparatus is functioning reasonably well for them, to build up habits of good-use *before* physical problems develop for them? The finest teachers and the most promising students find it hard to take seriously matters that are not directly connected with the finding and sounding of the notes on their instruments.

The Alexander teacher, generally a non-specialist in performing skills, but a specialist in background physical states, can often see more clearly what needs to be changed than the performer who is engaged in his exacting, attention-consuming task. The reason why he can, in his own field, use such absolute terms as "use" and "mis-use" is because he is describing basic states: posture- and tension-patterns in potential rather than in application. (Mathematically speaking, *Use* to the power of 0 will always equal unity.)

Yet there is a likelihood (which you may not choose to call a danger) that the Alexander teacher, as well as the dedicated instru-mentalist, will see things from a pure—almost too pure—point of view. Having had many lessons myself, and having been to concerts with Alexander teachers (including my wife) I am aware how they, and even I, have become sensitized to observe varieties of misuse which would never worry the uninitiated. The way a soloist walks on to the platform, slouches over his instrument, twists and writhes as he strives to put over the message, seems to call out to us for remedy. Can we assume that *all* performers would gain if their, not strictly functional, idiosyncrasies of behaviour were ironed out? Pictures of medieval singers show tense, strained throats; some modern singers knowingly reproduce the appearance and, presum-ably, the sounds that went with it. Perhaps some sounds can't be produced with the freed neck which is the starting point of all Alexander work? Paganini's bowing "was accompanied by such strange body movements that one could expect at any moment the upper body would detach itself from the lower". Is there not a possibility that the demoniac quality of his performance was enhanced by the non-resolution of internal tensions, and by the fact that his body was indeed a battleground for physical and mental forces? Though in the last 50 years, fashion has swung towards a restrained

and impassive sort of platform behaviour, Leonard Bernstein (as he
himself has said) is still paid to have epileptic fits in public, and pop
singers are still encouraged to advertise their emotions in actions.
Their admirers might reasonably suggest that, in the context, misuse
has become good-use; for the quality of their performances would
certainly change if they were sorted out Alexander-fashion.

It is clearly difficult for mature and established performers to
abandon attitudes which have become built in to their platform
characters over the years. Some may sense a risk in changing the
relationship (imperfect though it may be) between themselves and
their instruments—fearing the setting-up of a chain of unknown
consequences, as a husband or wife may fear consequences if a
psychiatrist should reveal to them weaknesses in a marriage which
they have so far concealed even from themselves.

But I am only playing devil's advocate in half-hearted fashion.
For I am sure that most practising musicians could benefit from the
technique. The enthusiasm shown by teachers, students, and performers supports this view. Musicians (if they are not too firmly
fixed in their ways) are particularly well-placed to benefit.

On a purely physical level, pianists and string players are by their
training conditioned to find the technique acceptable. They are
already versed in delicate muscular skills involving keen perception
in matters of co-ordination and precise forward-planning. There is
no need to impress on the string-player the need for economy of
movement (for instance, in string-crossing) or for perfect smoothness
of action in the bow-change, which is so like the smooth, almost
imperceptible change-over from outbreath to inbreath.

The enthusiasm with which the player who is already on the
upward path accepts and digests the technique springs from the fact
that it speaks to him of things that he already, imperfectly, knows.
Why, then, does he need a teacher? The answers would be much the
same whether you were questioning the need for a violin teacher or
for an Alexander teacher. (There is even a book called *Teach Yourself
The Violin*; but I have never met anyone who taught themselves any
stringed instrument without skilled help.) These main reasons are:
First, because the activities involved are complex; unless we have a
detached observer to hold the balance of attention for us, we are
almost bound to neglect some vital factor or to concentrate on one
aspect of performance at the expense of another. *Second*, because
discrimination in musical sounds or in physical states can only be
acquired by degrees, and cannot be conveyed in advance by words.
For this reason, we cannot, in early stages, *know* the way ahead. We

need the external guide who can see the whole course, and can steer us past blind turnings that seem to be leading the right way, but will in fact get us nowhere. *Third*, because we have a psychological blindness to our own defects, quite good players will develop mannerisms and defects which can be glaringly obvious to others, and which they could notice well enough in someone else's performance. For the player who can stand the shock, the tape-recorder may be of use, holding up a cruel mirror that reflects reality rather than the imagined ideal. But there is no recorder that reflects the shades of physical change in the human body. And *fourth*, because, in music and in physical states, there are many truths that lie beyond words. That is why there is a limit to what can be learned from older books, and is also why the Alexander teacher can come to play an increasingly important part in the training of the complete musician.

TWENTY-TWO

Research at The Royal College of Music
by Dr Wilfred Barlow

IN RETROSPECT IT often seems inevitable that certain developments should have taken place when they did: but in reality a huge part is usually played by chance. The reception of new ideas has always tended to be grudging or hostile, apart from those happy few whose work already has great prestige. An anecdote about J. J. Waterson is a good illustration—it was originally told by Wilfred Trotter and printed in my book *Knowing how to Stop*.

J. J. Waterson was an engineer who interested himself in mathematical physics and in 1845 he wrote a paper on the molecular theory of gases which anticipated much of the work of Joule, Clausius and even Clerk-Maxwell. The only contemporary judgement on the paper that survives is that of the referee of The Royal Society, to whom it was submitted. He said: "The paper is nothing but nonsense." What Waterson might have accomplished if he had had the recognition and encouragement upon which his genius seems to have been unusually dependent is beyond conjecture. He did not get them. His work lay in utter oblivion for 45 years, and he himself lived on disappointed and obscure for many years.

Wilfred Trotter, commenting on this story, wrote:

This little story must strike with a chill upon anyone impatient for the advance of knowledge, and especially upon such as are inclined to suppose that the use of the scientific method automatically follows on the possession of a scientific education. The mind delights in a static environment and if there is any change to be itself the source of it. Change from without, interfering as it must with the sovereignty of the individual, seems in its very essence to be repulsive and an object of fear. A little self-examination tells us pretty easily how deeply rooted in the mind is the fear of the new, and how simple it is when fear is afoot to block the path of the new idea by unbelief and call it scepticism, and by misunderstanding and call it suspended judgement. Let us hope that the genius of the future will find an intellectual environment where even his most revolutionary ideas will be planted in a nourishing soil and bathed in a genial air.

In 1949, even though the Alexander Technique had been outstandingly vindicated by the winning of the court case against the South African government, the "soil" in the UK was far from nourishing for it, and there was very little "genial air" around for it. Alexander himself was in his declining years and, like Waterson, was disappointed: his personal writings at that time show "a long-gathering impulse of despair". I myself had seen a medical career totally destroyed by the South African case, even though in every respect our evidence had been vindicated.

It was in such an atmosphere of hostility and depression that chance began to play a very fortunate part. When it was clear that orthodox medicine wished to have nothing to do with me because of the part I had played in Alexander's "victory", I had no alternative but to attempt to establish myself as a private medical practitioner, teaching Alexander's methods. Alexander himself had hoped that we would continue to work at Ashley Place, but there was no way in which, as a doctor, I could work in his employ and so a break had to be made. In 1949 I moved with my wife, Marjory, to rooms in Albert Court, close to the Albert Hall, gambling that with our very limited resources we would "make a go" of it, and finding ourselves very much between the devil and the deep, since neither Alexander nor the medical profession were prepared to be helpful. Fortunately, Marjory had always kept the thread of her Alexander practice going while she brought up our children and for several months we sat there hopefully, with only an occasional ring at the door. Then a young singer, Andrew Downie, who had heard of us indirectly in Paris, thought he would look us up. He had trained at The Royal College of Music, which, unbeknown to us when we set ourselves up in practice, lay only a short distance behind where we lived. After seeing us, Andrew decided to look into The Royal College of Music where he sought out one of his former professors at the Opera School, Joyce Wodeman. When she asked him how he came to be there, he said that he had just come from talking to two "Alexander" teachers who lived close by. "Oh, I've heard of Alexander," she said, "I read some of Alexander's books before the war and I have always wished to know more about it." So shortly afterwards she herself turned up at Albert Court and there was an immediate rapprochement between Marjory and this gifted professor, who in her turn encouraged a fellow professor, Joyce Warrack, to come and see us—two articles which they subsequently wrote are included here and Joyce Wodeman herself eventually trained to be an Alexander teacher.

It had soon become apparent to both of them that "Alexander" had much to offer to the musical profession and since they could no longer bear to see the way in which many of their students were misusing their bodies, they asked if they could send some of them to us for instruction—without any payment, I might add! But nonetheless very welcome.

By this time Clive Carey, who ran the Opera School along with Richard Austin, was beginning to take notice, and Sir George Dyson, Director of the College, was prepared to take the risk of letting me carry out research on a group of 50 of his students. The results of this research was set out in a paper which I subsequently read at The Royal College of Surgeons, and this, along with other research, eventually persuaded the medical profession that we were to be taken seriously—a switch of attitude which not long afterwards led to my being given a teaching hospital appointment in the NHS and to my present position as an NHS consultant. This particular paper was one which was of great importance to me personally, but also, I think, to the Alexander Technique since the "genial air" in which The Royal College of Music began to bathe us led not only to the confidence which comes from being accepted by people one respects, but to a snowball growth of the technique in the arts, at first spreading to the Central School (then located in the Albert Hall) and subsequently into many other establishments. The whole venture gave the Alexander Technique a new lease of life and one of my pleasanter pastimes used to be to trace back each new person who took it up to the first encounter with The Royal College of Music. Nowadays of course many many more factors have come in and there are many many more Alexander teachers advancing the technique in their own directions.

The essential rightness of Alexander's work was bound eventually to have made its impact, but "utter oblivion" was always a possibility in those early days—or almost as bad, a rather dreary meandering along as a fringe religion or as an adjunct to fringe medicine. My original paper on The Royal College of Music research was subsequently incorporated into a textbook, *Modern Trends in Psychosomatic Medicine*, and I have extracted from this the following report which was made by Joyce Wodeman and Joyce Warrack. Not only were there pronounced improvements in the students' bodily-use, but there was great success in a national music competition which eight of our students entered. Six of the eight entrants got through to the semi-finals and the winner was one of the group we had trained in the Alexander Technique. The actual photographs can be seen by anyone who is interested in *Modern Trends in Psychosomatic Medicine* (1954, Butterworth).

THE EXPERIMENT

Recently a group of 50 students under two professors from The Royal College of Music volunteered as subjects and they were re-educated by means of the Alexander Technique. Professor J. M. Tanner offered us facilities to assess alteration in use by means of Sheldon Somatotype-Photography. There are, of course, considerable limitations to assessing the manner of use by means of single photographs. A state of steady motion cannot be pinned down like a butterfly in a collector's cabinet. It would be fairly easy to give a misleading impression by a process of carefully selected photographs, and for this reason all the photography was carried out by Professor Tanner as a completely disinterested observer. He adopted the same procedure in posing the subjects as he adopts in his large-scale Somatotyping work.

The subjects had on average 37 lessons, although fewer than this might have been adequate. When possible I gave fifteen more or less consecutive daily lessons of half an hour and thereafter the students attended once or twice a week for a two to three month period for reinforcement and general guidance. All of the students except one gained in height, up to $1\frac{3}{4}$ inches, and the one exception was a student who maintained his original height but increased considerably in shoulder width. The results are given on page 99.

The Royal College of Music provided an excellent microcosm for the study of behaviour. Much of their work is taken up in presenting fortnightly performances of plays and operas, and there are regular examinations for various degrees: these activities provide plenty of scope for the generation of anxiety. The first students who came to me were originally picked out because of various specific troubles— poor movement and stage expression and minor medical disorders such as headache and low-back pain; but in the experiment a large number of "normals" were also sent. The professors in charge of the group were extremely experienced in their field and were examiners for the Associated Board of the Royal Schools of Music; their opinion was therefore a responsible one. The situation was excellent for investigating a new educational procedure, since to serve as a control there were numbers of other students who were not receiving

G

this single additional form of instruction. While a statistician might like to see it all planned out a little more formally, there is a lot to be said for using a living situation such as this in which there are recognized standards, and in which experienced teachers are quick to notice changes and have a shrewd idea of how quickly students can be expected to get on. The two professors prepared the following short report for me:

> In reporting on the progress of the 50 students we have sent you, it might be best first to outline our experience with other students before they came to you. We roughly classified students into three grades. First there were those with natural grace and freedom of movement and expression, who made good strides in their three-year training. Secondly, there were those who seemed to make no progress at all, and even deteriorated, during their training. Thirdly, there was a large in-between group, who, while not having any obvious gross handicap, never somehow quite made the grade. Dramatic and operatic work makes considerable demands on the student. The opera student these days needs not only a highly skilled vocal technique, but dramatic imagination and ability to express mood, emotion and character; he also needs musicianship, presence of mind and exceptional freedom and nimbleness of movement. During the training we gave them they did a great deal of mime and dancing, and in cases where specific muscular tensions were particularly noticeable they were given specific exercises.
>
> It was, however, our experience that during performance none of this training made a difference to deeply ingrained habit patterns. Habitual patterns of tension were not usually apparent to the student, and in most cases the student would strenuously deny the suggestion that he was tensing his body unduly. Our failures were all, without exception, over-tense when on the stage, either in a specific part of their body or generally. Any attempt on their part to relax could not be carried out specifically during performance, but was interpreted as a collapse of the whole body. By our ordinary approach we had reached a point where we saw that these tensions were responsible for the lack of progress of second-grade and third-grade students, but we were unable to deal with them. It was this problem that led us to try out the procedure you describe.
>
> It would take too long to go into individual case histories, but a few broad generalizations can be made.

1 In each case there has been a marked physical improvement, which was usually reflected vocally and dramatically. It was a revelation to discover that tricks of behaviour could be eliminated in a comparatively short space of time once the student learned to control his tensional balance from the head-neck region.

2 In all cases students since re-education are easier to teach, and can take and carry out stage directions with greater ease. The students seem to become aware of themselves in a new way. Each student reacted in a different characteristic way. For example, those who had been over-anxious to please authority discovered that they could be themselves with impunity, ceasing to be such model students, but becoming better performers.

One student, a girl hampered by angular stereotyped movements, and a curiously "spinsterish" quality of personality, has acquired considerable warmth and gracefulness. Another, with originally a very mediocre "drawing-room" voice, is now considered by her original teachers and critics to have developed the qualities of voice and personality that go to make a really great singer.

3 The time it takes to get results varies greatly between one student and another. The utilization of the approach depends largely on the student himself.

4 Eight of the 50 re-educated students entered last year for a singing prize which is competed for by women singers every four years. It is open to all amateur and professional singers under 30 years of age from anywhere in the British Isles, and is considered the highest achievement possible for students. The total entry was over 100. Of the eight students who entered six reached the semi-final, in which there were fifteen competitors. This is quite out of proportion to what one might expect.

5 In our opinion, this approach is the best means we have yet encountered for solving the artist's problem of communication and should form the basis of his training.

TWENTY-THREE

The Indirect Approach to Singing
by Joyce Warrack

ALL SINGERS, BY whatever method they study to achieve it, aim at a freely produced voice instantly responsive to the demands of interpretation. The instinctive reaction to any vocal difficulties inherent in such demands is to stiffen the neck and tighten the throat, or to seek comparative local freedom in the neck and throat at the cost of harmful habitual tensions in other parts of the body. Alexander's Technique for inducing self-awareness, and his insistence on the folly of attempting to control one set of muscles without reference to the total pattern of use in the person concerned, can therefore be of inestimable benefit to the singer.

Many of the great singing teachers seem to have foreshadowed this approach. Jean de Reszke would say: "Think for twenty minutes; sing for ten," and Vincenzo Vannini, in his book *Della Voce Umana* published in Florence in 1924, writes (my translation):

> Nature's means are essentially simple, it is only we who complicate matters with our pretentious attempts to be helpful. . . . All that the singer can do is to remain a spectator! He must cease to interfere and rather cultivate an attitude of intelligent laziness. . . . Nature has no need of our assistance. Leave the diaphragm to do its work; neither help nor hinder it *but leave it alone.* There is no need of special methods of breath control for singing, nor is there any lack of breath in the normally healthy human being. If there were he should hurry to see the doctor at once and then hope for the best!

Vannini considered singing as only slightly different from declamation or reading aloud—"It is a question of degree and getting accustomed to it. Once the new habit has been formed Nature imposes no obstacles." Alexander would have agreed; and only he, with his principle of "inhibition", has been able to supply the missing link that makes it possible for the individual to become conscious of his acquired misuse, and to provide for "a continuous change towards improving conditions by a method of *indirect approach,* under which opportunity is given for the pupil to come into contact with the unfamiliar and the unknown without fear or anxiety". Here is the crux of the matter for, as Alexander further points out: "People don't do what they feel to be wrong when they are trying to be right" (*The Universal Constant in Living*).

To teach the art of singing from this outlook is a stimulating if, at times, unnerving experience. Beyond the cool light of reason lurk the whirlwinds of urgent emotion and the instinctive fear of the unknown, seeming at present far beyond mental control—indeed, the word "control", not to mention "breath", will pitchfork the average pupil into a veritable strait-jacket of muscular madness. Knowledge of the technique, even if we do not always apply it, suggests the wisdom of attempting to take in an impression before trying to make one; and any intelligent pupil will see the point of this even if youthful eagerness may grudge the time involved in the process. Still——

Not to go back, is somewhat to advance,
And men must walk at least before they dance.

There are, according to Erich Fromm, four essentials for the professional approach to any art: discipline, concentration, patience and supreme concern. The first three provide the means of acquiring the necessary craft; the fourth can transform this into the realm of creative expression. To both craft and art Alexander's discoveries bring a new outlook, taking tradition as a starting-point, rather than as a sacred, crystallized memory; emphasizing the idea of living growth and change so that the singer, and later his listeners, can share in a vital and ever-fresh experience.

Anyone experimenting on these lines will inevitably be blazing his own trail, for there is a fundamental difference between this technique and those founded on the orthodox tradition of "Do as I do", in that the Alexander orders are concerned with basic principles rather than with exercising special parts. Nevertheless, diffidently and for what they are worth, I shall try to trace the steps that have led me to a tentative explanation of how and why all this really works.

First then, two questions: Who, or what, gives the orders? And who, or what, carries them out? I believe that seeking the answers to these questions, and observing the differing functions of the types of intelligence that make up the total pattern of our psychophysical being—and above all *noticing their time-ratio*—may lead us to the solution of a great many of our problems. Decisions, if consciously considered, are expressed as an order by the part of the brain that can reason and formulate the result in words. This is, however, a comparatively slow process—and it must also be remembered that *reason has no muscles* (nor for that matter have our emotions, much as they may be reflected in our everyday tensions!). Therefore, the only means of contacting the world outside ourselves is through our five senses and the amazing mechanism that knows how to regulate all our methods of circulation, our glands and internal organs (including the larynx and the vocal cords). It is this personal "computer" which, besides dealing with the in-built information that prevents us from committing hourly suicide, digests, for better or worse, the garbled instructions unconsciously fed into it by our ignorance and fear.

Compared to the leisurely pace of reason, instinct and emotion, those far-from-passive reactors to stimuli, work at lightning speed; and it is in recognizing and allowing for this time-factor that the possibility of control lies, with much saving of exasperation and strain. Here is the rôle for Vannini's "spectator", who should be able to watch the orders being carried out without interference. We were born breathing and yelling and, with a bit of luck, should be able to continue doing so with varying degrees of art and intelligence as long as we live. To the interpretative artist a vast number of stimuli have a direct impact on the emotions. Ideally, these impressions should be referred to reason instead of becoming the victims of blind instinct but, compared to other musicians, the singer is at a disadvantage in having to work with and through his own body—for no instrument is as unmanageable as the human organism in a panic.

Alexander's principles of inhibiting the immediate reaction, and of the indirect approach, are basic and all-important; therefore it is essential that both singing teacher and pupil should have personal experience as well as knowledge of his technique, and of its value in every facet of activity, before attempting to apply it to their particular field. Bad use cannot be modified; it must be stopped and replaced by something new and better. This entails a voyage of discovery. Does it also mean abandoning the traditional techniques associated with the singer's art? Not entirely; though, in the physical methods of voice-production and breath-control, it will be found that the Alexander orders, designed to induce the best possible relationship between the head, neck, torso and legs at any given moment, will make for an unconstricted throat and freedom for the lungs and thorax. It is interesting, too, to think in terms of the circulation of breath, with varying force according to demand, rather than of storing it up and squeezing it out like toothpaste. Conventional breathing exercises, which would seem to be an attempt at direct control of a specific function, rather than maintaining the conditions that would make this possible, can be replaced by Alexander's "Whispered Ah", where attention is focused primarily on the *orders* and not the *breathing*.

On the other hand, skills have still to be learnt: scales, arpeggios, ornaments, etc., as well as the music and words. Above all, their meaning, and the composer's intentions, must be understood and pondered; and here de Rezske's injunction "Think for twenty minutes" (for many, many twenty minutes!) holds the key, for we must not only know what has to be said and sung but how we wish it to be expressed. Once this is completely clear in our minds, it can be handed over with confidence to the swift-working machinery that transforms our thoughts and desires into the field of action. Re-education will indeed require patience and time (though a singer's training by whatever method is a lengthy process), but the resulting ease and command of his nerves, as well as the flexibility and living quality in the voice, will be ample recompense, giving the maximum result with the minimum physical exertion. Effort will have found its true rôle as objective attention and concentration.

From this it is only one step to the art of interpretation. Here the stimuli have to be evoked consciously and the characters, thoughts and emotions recreated in the light of the composers' and writers' vision. The secret is passively to "let your imaginary forces work". The "spectator" will find that each character, and in closer detail each mood, either in an operatic rôle or, more subjectively, in a lyric set to music, will impose its own manner of use. To his amazement these emotions and characteristics will seem to have an existence of their own and to be *teaching him*, though they are making use of his body. If, during the period of study, he is able to maintain his "watching brief" and confine himself to noting and inhibiting wrong and unnecessary muscular tension, he will achieve an interpretation "in depth" with each part fulfilling its own function in just relationship to the whole. To this intensely satisfying experience the Alexander Technique provides the key.

TWENTY-FOUR

Tension and the Actor
by Joyce Wodeman

BEFORE I CAME across the Alexander Technique I used to be aware of bad habits of use in some of my drama students without understanding what was wrong or what to do about it. I don't mean so much awkward or ugly mannerisms, for most young people who hope to perform publicly are sufficiently conscious of themselves to be able to get rid of these superficial bad habits. I mean rather those deep-seated tensions and constrictions that one sees to be typical of the person's activity as a whole and of which he is largely unconscious: in other words, what in Alexander terminology is summed up as someone's "manner of use".

As I say, I was not unaware that these habits were there and that that they were preventing students from doing their best; but since I had no clear idea of their cause, still less whether this cause was under the person's control, it did not seem feasible to try to eradicate them. One had to be satisfied with trying to minimize the effects. I have since found that I was not alone in being somewhat helplessly aware, in those one is teaching, of tensions that seem too much a part of their "character" to alter. Many teachers of drama, singing and music have admitted to a similar experience, and no doubt it is also encountered in the teaching of most kinds of sport and skill.

This half-acknowledged feeling of frustration in my professional work was what first attracted me to Alexander's teaching, for I believed I saw there the key to the problem of fundamental rigidity and tension. For me, Alexander's work has meant—as well as personal benefit—the ability to perceive much more clearly how my students are interfering with themselves when they act, and also (most encouraging of all) the knowledge that a method exists for freeing them of these interferences if they like to take advantage of it.

What form does bad use normally take in my students and how does it affect their acting? Basically, of course, it takes the same form as in all of us—pulling back the head, pulling in the back, hunching the shoulders, stiffening the arms and legs, and so on. These habits are harmful to everyone, but they can be a particular handicap to an opera singer. A performer who has to act as well as sing is subjected to numerous demands on his attention; as well as the musical exigencies (few singers, for example, approach their top notes without a certain apprehension), there is the "business" of the play to keep in mind and the need to match gesture and movement to the music and the words. All this means that a good opera singer must be exceptionally alert, with a freedom of movement which is nevertheless completely under control; rigidity or unconscious constrictions are the worst possible conditions for a good performance. Unless there is easy command of voice and body—a general fluidity—the singer is liable to give a wooden, strained impression and to falter at a critical moment.

Acting in opera also makes a further demand that distinguishes it, I think, from acting in a play—at least, in a modern play. The aim of many playwrights today is to convey feeling and situation "realistically", i.e. through those clipped asides, nervous little gestures and slight changes of tone that often betray our emotions and reactions in real life. It can be very effective—but this style of acting is completely unsuitable for opera. In this medium, instead of compressing expression, the student must learn to "extend" himself. A gesture to accompany an avowal of love sung over several bars must be a large, slowly unfolding one. In my experience, students whose manner of use is poor, and who have developed a lot of tension in the arm-shoulder-neck region, find this kind of "extended expression" very difficult to manage. The plays we use in class are mainly those—Shakespeare and Sheridan, for instance—which call for this expansive, declamatory style of acting; but one realizes again and again that no amount of "showing-how" or instruction imposed from outside can achieve a desired result as long as a person's deepest habits are pulling against it.

What I have said will by now, perhaps, have given you a broad idea of the benefits that students (the receptive ones, at least) derive from Alexander lessons. The clenched, tight underlying condition begins to yield; the student visibly "opens up", losing the stiffness and rigidity that made him clumsy, ungainly and uncontrolled in his actions. However, let me try to be more specific about the results.

First of all, students undoubtedly become more teachable—more able to take in what one is saying, and more able to accept criticism without feeling that they have "failed" abysmally when told they are doing something wrong. The main reason for this is, I think, that lessons in the technique shift one's centre of concern from trying to be "right" to thinking of all one's activity as a process that has become ill-directed in some respects, but can be put right by conscious re-direction. The change of attitude in students is often very marked;

from being over-confident or over-anxious, they come to accept more humbly the fact that we are all at fault in our different ways, but have it in our power to change if we are ready to be objective towards ourselves. As a first step this must involve learning how to stop doing the familiar thing (which feels right because it is so familiar that it is no longer conscious in order to experiment with and experience something new). This realization that one can always inhibit and re-direct brings a sense of security; what fundamentally makes for fear of criticism and discouragement in all walks of life, I am sure, is the pernicious idea that "being right" is the only criterion and that if one is "wrong" one has flopped as a human being!

Freedom from obsession with right and wrong has another effect—a rather amusing one, sometimes. The "too good" student, the sort who is over-anxious to please teacher, tends to become not nearly so "good" after a few Alexander lessons! And this is certainly better for them in their careers, because the dependent, placatory type of person never makes a good actor. While there is an element of impersonation in acting, it has to be creative, born of one's own perceptiveness and originality.

One finds in students who respond well to Alexander lessons a steady growth in awareness of their own habits and manner of use. This too contributes to better acting for inner and outer powers of observation are very much bound up. Perhaps a story will explain what I mean. In a particular production of *Rheingold* the problem of maintaining the illusion of the three maidens disporting themselves in the Rhine was achieved by strips of gauze, suitably lit, stretched across the stage, while the three maidens (only visible to the audience above the waist) paddled themselves about in low trolleys controlled by their feet. The swimming illusion was splendid but a difficulty cropped up when each maiden in turn had to slither off a high rock into the water and swim away. It was obvious that two of them, by unconsciously jerking their heads back as they landed on their trolleys, had landed on something extremely hard; the third, who had lessons in the technique, was able to control this "natural" reaction and looked as if she were slipping into water. The producer was delighted with the third maiden and told the others to copy her, and then added "Notice, she tips her head *back* when she reaches the trolley"! This pinpoints, I think, the problems in both reaching and learning. We can generally see whether a movement is satisfactory or not. It is when we venture into diagnosis that we are conditioned by our unconscious habit patterns.

As an experiment in observation, I sometimes get the class to walk across the room, one by one, and pick up a light chair. Those who are watching soon begin to notice how the "guinea pig" is already preparing, halfway across the room, to pick up a chair whose weight is quite unknown to him! As we go through the class, the students become conscious in themselves, too, of this anticipatory tensing-up.

I should like to emphasize finally that no form of teaching, not even the Alexander Technique, can make a good opera singer out of someone who does not possess the voice, musical ear and potential acting talent. What the technique can do—and does do to a striking extent in some cases—is to awaken the student to how he is strangling his natural capacity and provide him with the means-whereby to stop doing so.

Moreover, the student gains something that can be of immense value if he or she eventually attains the higher reaches of the profession where pressure and competition are gruelling—the conscious "know-how" for picking oneself up and finding the way back to one's true form if some accident or crisis temporarily upsets it.

TWENTY-FIVE

The Alexander Technique and the Actor
by John Gray

BOTH ACTING AND the Alexander Technique seem to be endlessly fascinating subjects for discussion, at least amongst those who know something about them, but they are both notoriously difficult areas. What is a good actor? It is almost impossible to define and perhaps in the final analysis it is merely one that you like. What is a good Alexander experience? Just as difficult to say, and not necessarily always one that you might like, for here you are contending with two of the strongest forces in life: feelings and habits, and a good feeling isn't necessarily a freeing of oneself from a harmful habit. The Alexander experience can mean quite different things to different people. It depends on HOW one has been interfering with the efficient natural use of the whole psychophysical mechanism as to what the "freeing" of that mechanism from misuse means to the subject, and as there are an infinitely variable number of ways of misusing oneself so there are an infinite number of new experiences that can be gained through being re-educated into improving use. However, in both areas there are perhaps certain generalizations that can be made and I'd like to examine some of them where the two fields come together.

An Actor's Training
Whether one's approach to acting is through Stanislavsky and all that that entails in the way of self-analysis, "living" the character, and developing the imagination, or whether one follows the seemingly simpler dictum of Noel Coward to "stand up, speak up, and don't bump into the furniture", whether one's motivation is Truth or the pay packet at the end of the week, one still needs the means to be able to work in these different ways. The freeing of the body is a prerequisite and directly connected to the freeing of the mind in order to release and develop the flow of imagination. Security in one's new good habits of thinking and use of the body, with all that that includes in the way of more reliable feeling and appropriate reaction, is essential for one's study of a character and ability to express the truth gained through study. Nor is it less important to know HOW to stand up, HOW to speak up, and HOW not to bump into the furniture.

In an actor's training he is expected, in the course of a couple of years, to absorb many techniques and develop in various areas. The clear idea of a reliable and sturdy "body-image" is vital if he is not to become over-absorbed and bogged down in one or two areas at the expense of a clear, balanced view of himself and his progress. There is little point in having the most vivid imagination in the drama school if you don't have the ability and means of expressing that imagination. There is no point in being the most expert fencer if the voice is constricted, inaudible and lacking in tone. Your singing might be heavenly but if you move like a robot it detracts from the total effect.

From my own experience when a drama student I know the confusion and agony of playing a part such as Othello: having to think of how I was using my voice, how to move in a suitably characteristic noble manner, how not to let my native dialects creep in to my newly-acquired standard English which was more suited to the Shakespearean verse; and was I getting the rhythm of the verse right, was I making the most of my small stature in this grand rôle for which I was naturally so unsuited, etc.? Not to mention having to sustain a very demanding rôle throughout the evening and then, over a number of performances, having to remember this sizeable part, giving the right cues to my fellow actors and making the right moves, and above all creating the right impression in all the various aspects of my technique to be certain that all my teachers would see I'd improved that term. If I had had a strong central core of awareness of myself into which I could absorb these techniques and necessary changes, and a more reliable means of bringing about these changes and improvements, instead of trying to force them upon a basically misused instrument, I have no doubt that I would have been happier and could have made better and faster progress. Working through the Alexander Principle allows this strong central core of awareness to develop and it becomes a checking point to which one can return after going off at a tangent or over-emphasizing any aspect of one's technique. It is not only a vital centre from which to work, but a steadying base and a framework for progress; and in no way a constricting framework but a freeing means of learning and absorbing new areas of technique so that in performance the actor can forget about his voice, speech, movement, fencing, singing, dancing, etc., and just get on and do it, secure in his means of performing. This all presupposes a great stability on the part of the actor in his new improved manner of use and so it is desirable that the actor approaches this side of his training as early as possible, ideally as a kind of pre-training, for the more immured he is in his misuse habits the more he will have related his development of his needed techniques to these harmful habits and the more difficult it will be to change them, as what dubious security he possesses will be through this misuse.

To add to all the other difficulties the young actor is expected to be coping with a vigorous training programme just at the time of life when all kinds of other major problems are being thrown up: the late teens and early twenties when he is having to face problems regarding his sexuality, possibly leaving home for the first time, managing on limited finances etc., so any steadying influence that allows him to develop greater awareness and self-knowledge, self-confidence and control is to be encouraged, and in this the Alexander Technique fits the bill.

Inhibition

The concept of Alexander Inhibition is often a confusing idea to the young actor. He feels that to say "no" to his reaction to a stimulus is going to seriously interfere with his spontaneity, the precious freshness in his work that is usually attractive and makes it convincing to the audience; and indeed it probably will in the early stages of his Alexander re-education. This, however, is because he has the wrong idea of what is true spontaneity. His habitual, automatic, reflex reaction, which he thinks to be spontaneous, is probably nothing to do with the appropriate reaction. Indeed it is probably a complex set of bad habits, accumulated over the years for a million different reasons, which are actually positively preventing him bringing about such a reaction. It might *feel* right to react in a certain manner, but quite often the audience is not impressed—to them it is quite obviously either an over-reaction, perhaps a lack of reaction, or even a positively wrong reaction to the situation or stimulus, and it is usually thought of as "bad acting" or "over-acting".

Alexander's "Inhibition", by making it possible not only to free the mechanism but yet have a conscious control of it, allows a more appropriate or desired reaction to be brought about, with the result that the actor has none of the irritation of suspecting that he may be reacting unsuitably (yet he does not know how to react in any other way): he knows he has the approval of his audience. The anxiety which might stem from a past bad experience or from an unreasonable anticipation of all the things that could go wrong will have been replaced by his Alexander awareness and control: he can stop such anxiety from coming between his intention to act and the actual action. He is more able to "hold" his audience, guide their feelings and coax their reactions into the right areas, using his talents towards a mutually enjoyable and satisfying result. "Inhibition", in this sense, frees rather than inhibits him.

Personal Traits of the Actor

More and more it seems the theatre wants to exploit an actor's particular peculiarities, especially in this day of television characters and personalities; there are so few good fat actors around that it is difficult to suggest to them that they slim for the good of their health as they might well not work so often. The Alexander teacher sometimes hesitates to help take away from an individual these traits, however harmful they might be, if the actor's living has been made through his exploitation of, say, his lack of co-ordination, his speech defect, or whatever, and then the choice has to be made as to whether to relieve this problem which seems to be so professionally useful or whether to leave it alone. But at least the individual now has the choice, before this he probably had no means of changing things reliably; and even if he chooses to hang on to his oddities, through his Alexander lessons he will at the very least prevent the effects of such habits being quite so harmful and might well change radically for the better in other areas. In the long run, however, I suggest that change is the only really viable approach, for apart from the sheer boredom to both actor and audience of his playing the same type for a whole lifetime, even bearing in mind the audience's love of the familiar, surely it is better and more interesting to all concerned if the actor is given the means to continue both to do the familiar and yet build up a reasonable norm of good-use of himself from which he can venture both as an actor and as a person into the other characteristics and reactions called for in a wider variety of rôles and situations. Very occasionally it might be better to simply leave well alone, as to make the required change would possibly, at least for a time, rob him of a confidence and security that have taken years to build up; and so perhaps his livelihood. Fortunately, however, most artists are only too aware of their insecurities and their need to change and develop stability and confidence: so on some worthwhile level or other they can usually appreciate the advantages of working in this way.

Learning, Playing and Sustaining a Rôle

The more secure the actor is in his new good-use patterns and awareness that he has built up through his Alexander lessons the more directly he will be able to apply it to his work so that however grotesque and misused the character he is portraying needs to be, it is unlikely to detract from his awareness of himself. He won't mix up the misuse of the body brought in to aid his characterization with the more stable and reliable good-use patterns he has developed through his Alexander work. Indeed his new good use will help him to misuse himself without harm, for it is the unconscious habitual misuse that really does the damage; we all have to do things to ourselves that would be potentially harmful if they become incorporated into the unconscious habitual pattern but are no great threat if one is very aware of one's manner of use. Even if the actor is not completely secure in his new, better way of using himself—for the necessary change to gain reasonable security can often take some time—at least he should have gained in some lesser time the means of getting back to a balanced state of rest after the periods of gross misuse often required in performance; a long run playing Quasimodo is not going to encourage him to incorporate into his habitual manner of use the subtle hint of the hunchback.

Playing the same rôle for a long period offers other pitfalls besides an over-identification with the character being played. The means of learning the part and building up the character in the first place are here very important. If the actor stumbles haphazardly upon the characterization or learns the lines parrot-fashion or through a hard slog, it is less likely he will maintain a security in these things than if he had worked from the start through a clear awareness of certain aspects of himself called into play during the rehearsal period. His technique will be built on firmer ground than merely trusting instinct and effectiveness, which tends to get dulled as a long run progresses and one forgets why one did such a thing, and, worst of all horrors to the actor, one forgets one's lines! This last problem commonly seems to get worse as one gets older, but if one's means of concentration are the Alexander means, a consciously controlled and developed awareness and attention to the whole psycho-physical mechanism, then the problem is less likely to arise than if one has thought of concentration in the more usual terms of needing to make a great deal of effort to get the part "under one's belt" through the drudgery of hours of repeating the lines till they go in and stick, with no attention to the means of learning and to what might be coming between the actor and his receptivity: i.e. an often gross misuse and interference in the whole psycho-physical mechanism.

"Resting" and Maintaining a Balanced Outlook

Great demands, both physical and mental, are made upon the actor both in work, and just as importantly, when out of work. He must be up to scratch at all times, for luck and timing are two of the greatest factors in his success. The precarious nature, financial and otherwise, of the profession has its good side, insisting that the actor constantly examines his motives and his values: can he afford to do such and such a thing, and if he decides he can then it is not so likely to be taken for granted and the simplest of actions can be a treat; more usually this precariousness, together with the excessive single-mindedness, or even ruthless ambition which seems necessary for success in this field, exerts a considerable strain on the individual over a period and can do untold damage. Feeling off-colour and looking so are a sure way to the Labour Exchange, so the actor's health is of paramount importance: he can't afford to be ill as he gets no salary if he can't work. Nor can he afford to be ill when he is out of work as it always seems to be at such times when the juiciest parts turn up. In his work he must be strong, able to cope with long hours of rehearsal and weeks of touring under Spartan conditions, playing demanding rôles often totally unsuited to his physical type, and yet always able to give the audience value for money and impress the producers sufficiently to employ him again. He must have the stamina to keep going for years without much reward and without becoming embittered and still be in good form when the golden opportunity arises, and as the success might be transitory, and the adulation rather meaningless, he will need the ability to adjust back into the more usual struggle after the "peak", having enjoyed the praise, invested the money, but not having gained a false idea of his own importance. He must also have the objectivity and strength of mind to direct his career into the sort of work that is going to further his success and yet be satisfying, and even turn down work if it seems to be the wrong job at this stage in his development.

The frustration of not being able to perform when unemployed is a constant strain. Most other artists can practise their skills even in the solitude of their own homes: the pianist can play, the singer sing, the painter paint, the writer write, even if no one is going to hear or buy their work; but the actor needs a job, a rôle, an audience, and usually other actors to work with, and yet even when he is able to perform there is no knowing that this job will be followed shortly by another in which he can consolidate the things he has just learnt through being employed. When "resting" his self-confidence is tested daily; unless he is very secure he feels he will never work again, often reaching the point where he is actually afraid to work yet desperately wanting to work and finding sometimes a spurious relief in being unemployed. Every audition is a time when he must impress and prove his worth, there are very few periods when he can simply coast along secure in his pay cheque at the end of the week. This constant testing is a constant strain so he needs a clear practical way of learning to release the excessive tension that is likely to build up, a fruitful channel into which his energy can flow when not needed for rehearsing or performing. The Alexander method is a reliable way of coping with these strained situations, so that his idea of life is level-headed and his approach to ill-health in general is preventive.

Conclusion
Most actors will need a method of conscious control and awareness to help them in both their lives and their work and the Alexander Technique most suitably fills the bill. In the recent past the approach to acting has been largely through "right thinking" and not enough through how to express such thinking. As the Alexander work frees the mechanism to become more expressive and sensitive in the work situation through a more stable and reliable manner of use in all activities, the effects of this are like the ever-enlarging ripple from a stone thrown into a pond. Any therapeutic element there may have been in needing to act tends to get sorted out: whether it is an inability, guilt or awkwardness in expressing oneself, and therefore a tendency to hide behind another person's words or in another person's character, or if real life doesn't offer experiences that are sufficiently fulfilling and one finds more satisfaction in fantasy or imagination. In the re-educational process a pupil often finds the ability to express pent-up emotions or rid himself of hidden fears and stresses. A new self-confidence and clearer vision together with the contentment they seem to bring allows him to deal more appropriately with his problems and to accept them without their causing any irreparable damage to the personality or character. This change that the Alexander Technique brings about can often open the eyes of the actor to other interests so that he finds satisfaction in other fields and it is not uncommon for drama students (who now frequently study the technique) to realize earlier their shortcomings as actors or the likelihood of all the problems they will have to face and even change their ideas of pursuing a career in the profession. Whether or not it is a good thing to take away some part of their "drive" at this early stage, however suspect this element of their ambition, through helping them to release themselves from their personality problems, is perhaps the subject of another article, but to

my mind, as an actor, the sooner one's eyes are opened to the full meaning of a career in the theatre, the horror and the heartbreak as well as the enormous attractions, the better for all concerned. There is no doubt that acting can be a useful therapy but it surely is preferable to gain stability from the realization of one's true self, fully expressed in a real-life situation. There are enough rôles to play in everyday life without being constantly muddled by the doubly-deep area of having to play rôles professionally in order to find any kind of satisfaction for feelings and emotions. In short, get sorted out first and thereby find out your true motives for pursuing a career in acting. Possibly the most difficult dilemma to an actor is that he so often doesn't know if he is *acting* or really *experiencing* his feelings.

Lucky and rare is the actor who is 100 per cent fit and fulfilling most of his career, who doesn't meet problems with his breathing, voice, movement or the deeper areas already discussed, who is in fact so naturally well co-ordinated that he doesn't need to think frequently about his instrument of work—his whole psycho-physical mechanism. To be able to take full advantage of all the wonderful opportunities offered by this totally dotty profession in the way of helping a personality to develop through imagination and curiosity and confidence in one's ability requires exceptionally fortunate circumstances. The Alexander Technique at its most basic level is there to help as a practical positive means to achieving such development and satisfaction in work and life and relationships by eliminating over-work in the body and over-tension in movement and action as well as static rigidity, and encouraging a profitable "flow" of energy through an on-going, improving, dynamic manner of use.

APPLICATIONS

SCIENTIFIC

TWENTY-SIX

Mr Alexander's Use of Scientific Method
by Professor A. E. Heath

What Scientific Method is
Scientific Method consists essentially of two steps:

1 The collecting and critical testing of a body of facts, and
2 The systematizing of those facts, by means of appropriate ordering conceptions, into an intelligible whole: "Science is an attempt to render intelligible bodies of facts in any fields"—(Sir Percy Nunn).

These two steps which constitute scientific method are like the process of walking by placing first one step and then the other forward. Thus, once the primary facts in any domain of human experience have been observed, they are then ordered. Such ordering directs us, in the process of verifying that order, to new facts. These, in turn, are susceptible of further ordering—and so on, in an endless series.

This analysis of the meaning of scientific method makes it clear that any field of experience (physical or mental or a combination of the two) can be treated scientifically: "What makes a study scientific is not the things it deals with, but the way it deals with those things" (Sir J. A. Thompson).

Mr Alexander's Use of Scientific Method
Step 1. The beginning of Mr Alexander's work was entirely *empirical*. That is to say he discovered (or rather, re-discovered and greatly emphasized) the importance of the head-neck relationship in the erect human posture. What, however, was new in Alexander's critical checking of the facts concerning this head-neck relationship was the hitherto unrecognized fact that extreme difficulty is experienced when we try to adopt a correct posture. It is easy to recognize the *end* to be achieved but very hard to develop the *means* of achieving it.

Still at the level of factual investigation, Mr Alexander developed a special technique for ensuring head-neck posture, and discovered that in doing so many kinds of malfunctioning of the body-mind organism were lessened or removed. This factual basis to Alexander's work makes it essential, for its judgement or assessment, to examine the technique in actual practice.

Step 2. The facts that Alexander collected clearly called for an explanation. To be understood or made intelligible they must be systematized by some appropriate and effective ordering conception. Broadly speaking the conception, which brought systematic order in to the body of facts disclosed by Alexander's special technique, is that of regarding the whole process as a method of conscious and deliberate inhibition of habitual postures and tensions which the strain of living in civilized societies has superimposed upon man's original achievement of an upright position. Thus the neck muscles which have become habituated to over-tension drawing the head back, have to be deconditioned to such tension before the correct head-neck position can be assumed. The difficulty lies in the fact that what we are habituated to *feels right*, and the first attempt at conscious adjustment *feels wrong*. Mr Alexander's technique is simply a mode of procedure which is designed to overcome this practical initial difficulty.

Step 1 again. With this ordering of the facts once established, the next step was to go back to the empirical factors disclosed by the results of successful technique. It was found that a great variety of other types of malfunctioning could be adjusted to more effective functioning. The test by results may be called "operational verification". The variety of these results is not surprising in view of the fact that the body-mind is one organic unity.

At this stage it became evident that Mr Alexander's purely educative work, besides being of practical therapeutic value, was in line with the work of other men of science who, like Sir Charles Sherrington, stress the central integrative function of the nervous system, both voluntary and reflexive.

Step 2 again. Alexander's technique for achieving the step from knowing *what* to knowing *how*, has other theoretical bearings. It is clearly related to John Dewey's philosophy of instrumentalism as applied to human behaviour, both individual and social.

Recently an English philosopher, Professor G. Ryle of Oxford, has put forward an analysis of knowing which has a real similarity to Alexander's distinction between knowing the means whereby such ends can be achieved. Professor Ryle says the maxims of a practice presuppose knowing how to perform it. "Rules, like birds, must live before they can be stuffed" (G. Ryle, "Knowing How and Knowing That").

In short, Alexander's technique may have a very important bearing in the future on educational practice. What Dr Barlow calls "kinaesthetic re-education" may have repercussions even in academic studies.

TWENTY-SEVEN

Use and Misuse in Evolutionary Perspective
by N. Tinbergen, F.R.S.

(An Alexander Memorial Lecture given in November 1976)

Defining the Problem

Since I am not an Alexander teacher myself, have not watched more than a few members of the guild at work, and have been a pupil for no more than three years, it would be presumptuous if I were to pronounce on the technique itself, how it works, and why it works. *That* it can have strikingly beneficial effects I can, like many others before me, testify on the basis of changes I have observed in quite a number of my acquaintances and in myself.

What I feel more competent to talk about is a biological aspect of the Alexander Principle that has so far been treated rather lightly: that of the genesis of misuse. What causes, or has caused, those patterns of faulty posture and movement that Alexander teachers are trying to correct, often with such striking success?

That misuse in its many forms is widespread at least in our western societies cannot be doubted, except by those who do not pay attention to how other people stand, sit, and move. What is more difficult to judge is whether misuse is a relatively recent phenomenon, or whether perhaps all preceding generations have had just as defective use, which remained unnoticed until Alexander called attention to it. The question is of considerable importance for our understanding of what "Alexandering" really does. Several authors claim that misuse is largely a response to modern living conditions, to a changed style of life. If this were true, we would have to do with a relatively recent, non-genetic deterioration (for genetic change of this magnitude would take an infinitely much longer time). But other authors interpret misuse in a different way; they assume that Man's evolution as an upright walking, bipedal primate has not yet been completed; they claim that our use is not *yet* perfect, and that, as Alexander himself suggested, conscious, rational education of our minds and bodies must "take over" from the genetic evolution that has moulded us until now.

If the first view is correct, then Alexandering is a method of correcting individually incurred damage; a re-education; a therapy. If we believe the second alternative to be true we assume, firstly, that as a species we are still on the way to better upright use; secondly, that we can predict the future course of our evolution; and thirdly, that we can help it along.

I feel that neither Alexander himself nor the various writers who have discussed his work have given sufficient attention to this problem, or, to the extent that they have done so, have skated rather lightly over it. At any rate it is not easy for the reader to gain an impression of what, if any, interpretation of the genesis of misuse a given author accepts. This is partly due to the fact that the various experts, each with his own intellectual background, express themselves in different ways, which has led to a certain degree of semantic confusion. Also, most authors (though not all) have given more attention to the therapeutical technique than to what we could call the biology of use and misuse. Yet a biological approach might help us in assessing more realistically the potential of the technique (for individually acquired misuse can be corrected much more easily than a genetic shortcoming).

Biologists are equally concerned with all organisms, and like to cast their nets wide. If I am therefore going to make a longish excursion into comparative biology I hope you will bear with me; I shall in the end return to the genesis of misuse.

Fitness

The biologist and (I am sure) many physicians look at "good use" as a special case of life processes that ensure fitness, adaptedness, the ability to do the right thing at the right time and in the right place; and at misuse as maladapted functioning. The expressions "fit", "adapted", "right"—referring to roughly the same thing—are biological shorthand for a statement about fundamental properties of living beings. They are not quite complete, for they refer to only one side of the coin. They do not mention (though they do imply) what the organism is fit *for*, what it is adapted *to*, what *is* "right". Something like an opponent, or a resisting, demanding force is suggested. And it is true that every organism has such an opponent, one it has to cope with competently on penalty of death. This opponent, continuously challenging, continuously threatening, is the organism's environment.

In order to see clearly what this means we have to realize that, to every living being, the environment is potentially destructive. There have, as far as we know, been two different lines of evolution of matter. One has led to the present non-living systems; the other to organisms. Though both have a common origin (the first life evolved from non-living matter), living and non-living things are now, after several milliard years, strikingly different. Stated very simply, non-living things proceed towards increasingly simple, increasingly probable, increasingly stable states. Living things do exactly the opposite: they develop in the direction of the complicated, the improbable, the unstable. I always like to illustrate this by a very simple example: if I release a stone in mid-air, it will fall, i.e. it will passively, meekly, obey the external force of gravity. But if I release a bird in mid-air, it will fly away; it "defies" gravity, or rather it counteracts it—it remains subjected to it; alive or dead, a bird has the same weight.

What the bird does is a special case of a "life process", typical of what all living things do. Gravity is only one "pressure" among many. Every organism faces a number of pressures and has to counteract each of them in one way or another if it is to stay alive. All animals have to take up food, water, oxygen; they have to defend themselves against temperature extremes, against parasites, against predators; they have to get rid of waste. Many of them have to do these things not merely on their own behalf, but also on that of their offspring. One can characterize living organisms by saying that they can stay alive and reproduce only by performing, with continuous vigilance, a tightrope act—so to speak a multi-dimensional tightrope act, in which they cope all the time with not one but with a number of environmental pressures. What is more, no two species live in the same habitat; even in the same terrain they have different "niches". So no two of them are faced with exactly the same pressures: e.g. each has its "own" kind of food and each is preyed on by its "own" predators. And different species meet these different pressures in different, but always in fitting ways.

One example must suffice to give at least a glimpse of adaptedness. It concerns the behaviour of a bird. It is more complicated behaviour than just flying, yet it is no more than a tiny part of the animal's total "equipment for success". Like many other birds the Black-headed Gull removes the empty shell of each of its eggs shortly after each chick has hatched. Unless the brood fails, each pair raises one clutch of three young a year. The removal of each empty shell involves no more than taking it up in the bill tip, flying between one and fifty yards or so away, dropping it, and returning to the nest. Each excursion lasts no longer than a couple of seconds, and the behaviour is shown during no more than the time taken by three trips, i.e. ten, at the most twenty, seconds each year. Yet those few seconds' absence are not negligible: predators such as crows, who are often hanging round gulleries, need only a few seconds for a "dash and grab" raid, in which they can steal an egg or a chick. One must assume therefore that the gulls take this risk because the response confers an over-riding benefit that outweighs the risk. And it has actually been shown that gulls' eggs that are laid out in the field, each with an empty egg-shell next to it, suffer much higher predation than eggs without such a "betraying" neighbour. The eggs of these gulls are beautifully camouflaged, having a khaki ground colour and many irregular dark dots. But once the chick has hatched, the broken egg-shell shows some of its white inside. The crows and other predators see this conspicuous white, and find the egg nearby. Egg-shell removal is therefore part of the defence of the brood against predators.

How sophisticated the gulls' behaviour machinery is for this one, seemingly so trivial, response becomes clear when we list some of the stimuli which make a gull remove an egg-shell. That the response is partly under internal control is revealed by the fact that the gulls remove egg-shells only in spring, some time before they actually lay eggs to a little after the young have hatched; in fact the graph of readiness to carry off egg-shells runs parallel to that of readiness to incubate. This suggests a hormonal factor, which, however, has not been identified, though prolactin seems a likely candidate. External stimuli to which the gulls respond were analysed by presenting incubating birds with dummies of egg-shells and scoring their responses. When this was done with dummies of different colours it was found that khaki and white dummies were removed far more promptly than those of any other colour. The main shape characteristic to which the gulls responded was "thin edge". Weight was also taken into account: shells that were much heavier than normal, empty shells, were taken up but then put down again (this prevents the gulls from "throwing away the baby with the bathwater"—a chick needs some time to work itself fully out of the shell even after the thin edge shows, and the parents' response to its weight prevents premature removal). Distance from the centre of the nest is an important stimulus: only shells very near the nest are removed, and with increasing distance the removal rate drops sharply. Finally, the shell is carried away soon after hatching, but not immediately. All these refinements of the gulls' responsiveness fit the requirements as imposed by the predators. Thus, when one presents eggs to wild crows with empty egg shells at different distances, they find fewer eggs the larger the egg–egg-shell distance is. Similarly the delay after hatching is useful because a newly-hatched chick, being wet and easily swallowed, is much more at risk than a fluffy, dry chick, which is far less attractive to a predator.

This is no more than a sketchy outline of some aspects of one simple adapted response. Yet it illustrates what I meant when I said that living is a multi-dimensional tightrope act—even if we look at behaviour that occupies only ten–twenty seconds of an animal's annual time budget. The response is a part of the (much more comprehensive) incubation system, and also part of the (likewise much more elaborate) anti-predator repertoire.

Many other studies have been made in which behaviour and environment are compared, and they are steadily enriching our picture of adaptedness, of the "fit" between on the one hand what the environment requires of the animal, and on the other what the animal actually does. For our purpose two general points are worth stressing.

Firstly, adaptedness of behaviour is not a matter of movement alone. As in "use" in the Alexander sense, structure is always equally essential; just as other life processes involve both structures and action, so movements are the result of *functioning structures*. Second, while I stress the conclusion that survival of animals, as of ourselves, depends on competence, on a sufficiently good fit between the subject's functioning and the environmental pressures, I have to emphasize just as strongly that competence is something quite different from perfection. No single animal or human functions perfectly. Two reasons for this are particularly obvious. As one would expect in organisms that have to cope with a number of pressures, the demands of one pressure may well, are almost bound to be, contradictory to those of another one. The animal meets such a situation with a compromise. We have already seen that the Blackheaded Gull times the removal of its egg-shell in such a way that the brood is not exposed too early (when the chick is still wet) but not too late either (when the chance of a predator seeing the conspicuous egg-shell grows). In the structure of living beings the compromises are often visible at a glance. The legs and feet of geese and gulls are striking examples. They are well suited to swimming—though not as well as the legs of, for example, a grebe. They are also good walking legs, but again no more than tolerably good—ostriches are far better walkers and runners. To use a technical analogy: an amphibious vehicle is neither a good boat nor a good car.

Another principle that can tempt us to say that an organism

performs less than perfectly (some biologists have even spoken of "construction errors") is "evolutionary restraint" or "historical load". We all, animals and ourselves, carry with us characteristics that evolved in our evolutionary past and that we are, so to speak, saddled with. For instance our own shoulder joint, which gives us such marvellous freedom of movement of the arm, was not originally evolved for the purpose of throwing a spear or even stones: it is of older origin and enabled our ancestors of twenty million years and longer ago to move through their forest habitat by "swinging" or "brachiating" from branch to branch. It so happens that we have put this "load" to good use, but if we would want to run on all fours, the shape of this joint (as well as later changes such as the evolution of hands) would make us cut a poor figure. Biologists who claim to find construction errors may well, by concentrating on single sub-systems, and on how they work now, have underrated the consequences of the "compromise" and the "historical load" principles.

To sum up this section: I have argued that equipment for fitness is (1) extremely complex; (2) extremely improbable; but (3) not merely, or randomly improbable: it represents one out of perhaps a million kinds of improbability, for it is adapted to a very specific environment. I stress these points because their combination demands, makes it imperative, that organisms be programmed for viable functioning. We have to consider how this programming is done.

Programming for fitness
If a species is to survive, a sufficient number of its young, i.e. one new reproducer for every adult that dies, must grow up, survive and reproduce. The growth of the equipment for this (and, as I said before, "equipment" embraces both structure and function—which in its turn includes of course movement, or use) is the result of two types of programming. Although these interact, support, and supplement each other, they must be sharply distinguished conceptually. Loosely worded they can be called "nature" and "nurture", respectively.

As to nature: when a new individual is conceived, it carries, in the nucleus of each cell, a system of giant molecules or genes, together called the genome, of which half has come from the father, half from the mother. The genome instructs the egg cell, and subsequent stages in the development, how to grow into an adult, and how to function. This is an infinitely complicated process, and science is only beginning to understand at least partially what actually happens.

To realize why development of organisms may well be the most formidable of all challenges to biological science it is sufficient to remember that, difficult though it is to understand how an adult animal functions, the development of these functions presents us with two additional obstacles. Growing, i.e. consistent and progressive change, adds the dimension of time to our problem; and (unlike a machine which need not function until it has been put together) a developing organism functions properly *while* it grows.

Every species has its own genetic endowment different from that of all other species. In the behavioural sciences we refer to this when we speak of innate differences between species. Within each species there are likewise (small) variations between individuals, and in fact no two individuals (except the members of identical twins or multiplets) are genetically exactly alike. Since in every species many more young are produced than survive until maturity, this inequality means that statistically, mortality will not be random; some individuals are bound to be fitter than others, and this is why natural selection, given less than perfection even of the best, can cause genetic evolution. It takes little reflection to realize that evolution-by-means-of-natural-selection is a huge trial-and-error game, played with the environment as the referee.

Nurture is a totally different, but in functional terms supplementary process. While an animal grows up, and in higher animals throughout life, an individual interacts with its environment, and changes as a consequence. The best known example of this individual "modification" (phenotypic as distinct from genetic change) is learning in its many forms, but the phenomenon is really much broader: e.g. we respond phenotypically to exposure to ultra-violet light by depositing dark pigment in our skin; our muscles are strengthened by use; exposure to infectious diseases can increase our resistance to them, etc. But the effects of phenotypic modification are not transferred to the genome, and so cannot be passed on genetically. Each generation has to acquire its modifications anew.

The changes that an individual acquires by modification are not random. Contrary to what psychologists have long believed, such changes are adaptive; in the natural environment they supplement, continue, polish what the genetic instructions are achieving. More: genetic and "experiential" programming interact with each other. Perhaps the most important aspect of this is that modifiability is itself under genetic control. There are two sides to this coin. Firstly, each species learns certain things very well, and other things not at all. An extreme example that comes to mind is that of some kinds of solitary wasps who travel back and forth between a burrow (in which they have deposited an egg and which they provision with captured and paralysed insects that have later to serve as food for the larva) and a hunting area where they capture the particular prey insects they need. On the hunting field they roam over a vast area in search of prey. Different preys may be found in widely different locations. For returning to the burrow they have to find their way with pin-point accuracy. Whenever they leave the burrow at the start of a new foraging trip, they make a careful "locality study", and it has been shown that it is then that they learn the position of the nest entrance in relation to landmarks in the surroundings (they can do this in as short a time as six seconds). But when they have captured a prey in the hunting area, they do not make a locality study, nor do they later return to the exact spot. Of course, with prey species that live scattered or are mobile, it is not necessary to remember where exactly a prey was found, but the point is: "How does the wasp know this?" Its genetic instructions have told it to learn this here and now, and not to bother elsewhere and at other times. Numerous examples of such "predispositions to learn" are now known.

The other side of the coin is that even selective non-learning has a positive aspect. Behaviour is often "environment-resistant" or "stubborn"; such behaviour (formerly called "innate") develops along genetically dictated lines "in defiance" of whatever attempts we might make to modify it. Even in our own species, genetically so "open minded" as far as behaviour is concerned that even now some scientists believe that we are infinitely modifiable, a great variety of behaviour traits are stubborn in this sense. For instance when walking we move our arms synchronously but in alternation. If we try to move right and left arm in different rhythms (e.g. right two versus left three), or in a two–five rhythm, we meet with enormous difficulties. I am told that two–three is a pattern that musicians and ballet dancers can learn, but with considerable effort. What a difference between this modest achievement and, say, the learning of a language!

We see, then, that genetic and phenotypic programming are inter-twined in many ways. The result is usually that it is possible to modify a behavioural or a structural aspect of the living machinery in certain directions and to a certain extent, but always within limits— ometimes wide, sometimes narrow. These limits vary from one species to another and, within species and even in one animal, from one behaviour to another. To come back for a moment to our arm movements: while it is difficult to modify the *rhythms*, it is very easy

H

to modify (increase or decrease) their *amplitude*. It is also easy to modify the *direction* of the swinging and to move them either in parallel, front-to-back planes (as in the British ceremonial military style) or in planes almost at right angles to the direction of marching (a Russian style). This incidentally illustrates how one can discover "stubborn" behaviours in Man: when a movement is "cross-culturally constant", i.e. virtually the same in all known cultures (as is true of smiling, crying and many other forms of non-verbal "language", which show only minor intercultural variations), it is largely programmed genetically. But if a movement varies consider-ably from one culture to another (as is the case with speech) the environment has obviously been influential. It is only slowly being acknowledged that our species, while clearly far more modifiable than any other, depends to a considerable extent on genetically given instructions, though the detailed analysis of our nature–nurture relationships has only just begun.

We are likewise far from understanding why the proportion of genetic and environmental or experiential programming differs so much from one species to another and from one behaviour pattern to another. But we do have indications that natural selection has to do even with subtleties of development, that they make functional sense. A butterfly, just hatched from the pupa, will at first hang motionless hooked on to the empty pupal skin, or on to the supporting twig. It will pump up its wings, then let them harden for a couple of hours, and will finally fly away, using its wings for the first time in its life. As far as we can see, this flight movement is fully competent right from the start. Of course it has to be, for a clumsily flying butterfly would at once be snapped up by the nearest songbird. Compare this with the relative incompetence of the walking movements of young dogs or kittens. Or with the "open-mindedness" of a young songbird who, shortly after fledging, is left to fend for himself. His flexibility is seen most clearly in the selection of food. If he had been rigidly instructed to feed on one particular kind of caterpillar, he would be very lucky indeed if he could earn a living, for each species of cater-pillar has a restricted habitat and, even more important, a hatching schedule that varies from one year to another. Natural selection, which forces a butterfly to be an accomplished flier from the very start, has forced the songbird *not* to base his choice of prey exclusively on genetic (innate) knowledge—not to know exactly what is good for him—but to start in an open-minded way, and then to learn by experience to go for what is edible and available. The result is that such a youngster can survive in a far wider range of habitats than he could if he were rigidly and narrowly instructed by his genes. These examples (and there are many more) give us at least an inkling of the reasons for these wide, and seemingly random variations in the "nature–nurture proportion" in behaviour programming; as far as we can see, this too is part and parcel of adaptedness.

After the general introduction, let us now turn briefly to what we know about our own evolution.

The Emergence of Man

In recent years our knowledge of the evolutionary history of Man has been growing by leaps and bounds. Of course, fossil and other remains being exceedingly rare, the picture is still far from complete, and the experts still disagree on many points. Yet a consensus of opinion begins to form on some aspects that are relevant to our theme.

Although some old pre-human remains have been found in Asia, there is now no doubt that the cradle of Mankind lies in Africa, in particular in east and south Africa. Our very remote ancestors were no doubt closely related to the forest dwelling "pre-apes" and moved mainly by swinging from branch to branch. The oldest fossil which reveals pre-human traits dates from *circa* ten million years ago, but since of this form (*Ramapithecus*) no more has been found than some teeth and jaw fragments, interpretation of this old ape is, despite the expertise of modern palaeontologists, uncertain. It is for instance not known whether it did, or even could, walk upright. Much more is known about forms appearing (approximately) five million years ago, and named by their discoverer, Raymond Dart, *Australopithecus* ("the Southern Ape"). All known Australopithecines seemed to have walked upright—a conclusion based on such things as the shape of the thigh bone, the placing of the *foramen magnum* of the skull and other particulars. There have undoubtedly been more than one type of *Australopithecus* and hence different streams of evolution, but only one survived to evolve in the human direction. The line of the giant *Australopithecus boisei* for instance, who was probably a vegetarian, is considered to have become extinct. The forms usually called *A. africanus* and/or *A. gracilis* are considered by many to be our real precursors. This line evolved larger brains than their predecessors, and, in later times (though still a couple of million years ago), began to use fire and to make crude tools. By this time the distinction between monkeys and apes was also quite sharp: monkeys were, and most of their descendants have remained, forest dwellers who alternated swinging with walking on all fours.

In this very gradual, to all intents and purposes gliding, process, of which we know only a few "snapshots", it is impossible to speak of sharply defined moments of change, just as we cannot say exactly at what moment a baby becomes a toddler. Nevertheless it is certain that our ancestors began to walk upright at least five million years ago—quite a respectable time span, which must have provided ample opportunities for the evolution of bipedal efficiency.

The change from brachiating to upright walking is so important because it was part of a much more comprehensive process: the invading, by our ancestors, of a new ecological niche. Lured into the open by the abundance of game on the east African savannah (and perhaps prodded by too much competition in the forest) they began to abandon their old haunts and became what is technically known as hunter-gatherers. It is supposed that, as in modern hunter-gatherer peoples, the men did most of the hunting, at least of large animals, while the women and children gathered such things as nuts and roots, and small animals such as insects, lizards, young birds etc.

Early Man could be successful in this venture because, being already social, he was capable of developing hunting-in-groups and so could overpower prey animals much larger than himself. Having control of fire, and being quite a competent tool maker he could also defend himself against the ferocious predators of the African plains. And finally, he was much more intelligent than any of the other animals. It has been said that the move to the plains, the habit of social hunting and the mastery of fire and tool making could not have evolved together if *Australopithecus* had not reached just the level of intelligence that he had. There are other social hunters on the African plains, such as the lion and the hyena, who have remained at the animal level. There are even monkeys, the baboons, who have adopted the hunter-gatherer life style. Yet they remained monkeys. Without Pre-Man's superior intelligence, he would probably never have held his own on the dangerous plains, and the plains game would have remained underexploited.

Once Pre-Man had chosen to go this new way, a process began that we know well from other animal groups. Whenever in evolution a species branches off from the original stock, it begins rapidly to adapt itself to its new niche. This involves a form of self-perpetuating change. For instance, by walking and running upright, early Man freed his hands for the making and using of tools and other forms of manipulation. But the more he adapted his hands to these tasks, the less suited they became for locomotion, and the more pressure was put on legs and feet to become more and more efficient locomotory organs. Likewise, tool making had become possible not only by the efficiency of hands, but also by the capability of the brain. But the more sophisticated the tools became, the more stringent grew the demands that both their manufacture and their use imposed on the brain. In other words, Pre-Man met a number of mutually and positively reinforcing pressures, which together spurred on rapid adaptation to the new niche. As a general rule, such adaptive evolution in a new niche does not slow down and stop until, within the limits set by "historical load", the best possible state of adaptedness to the new niche has been reached.

We know roughly how, once our ancestors had become hunter-gatherers, their further evolution proceeded. *Australopithecus* was succeeded by (probably evolved into) a much more human type, *Homo habilis* (who was, as his tool kit proves and his name indicates, "handier"). At least one million years ago, probably earlier, the even more Man-like *Homo erectus* had progressed so far that he could invade new areas of the globe: east and south Asia (where he was originally given the names *Pithecanthropus erectus* and *P. pekinensis*), Africa, and southern Europe (where one of his best investigated camping sites was discovered under the heart of the city of Nice). We know of *erectus* that he was a truly formidable hunter, who could kill elephants and wild horses. Approximately 100,000 years ago Neanderthal Man had appeared, for quite a time the most maligned of our ancestors, whose skeleton was at first completely misinterpreted. Now we know that he was already far advanced, was an extremely sophisticated tool maker (one population is known to have had at least 80 different kinds of tools), and, at least in some places, buried his dead. More: he lined the graves with conifer branches, and covered the corpses with layers of brightly coloured flowers, of which the study of their pollen has revealed the species. He lived in even more diverse habitats than *H. erectus*, and hunted down the very large and fierce mammals inhabiting the Arctic tundra. Most anthropologists believe now that at least some of the Neanderthal oppulations evolved into Cro Magnon Man, whose remains appear some 35,000 years ago and are indistinguishable from those of modern men. He too was an accomplished hunter, he lived in even more parts of the globe than his predecessors, survived harsh Ice Age conditions in various hitherto uninhabited regions, and he gave us an inkling of his artistic genius in the cave art of Altamira, Lascaux and many other caves.

Of special interest in our context is the fact that the fossil skeletons of these successive ancestors give us a good idea of the gradually evolving suitability of their legs, and in fact their whole build, for upright walking and running, and, even more to the point, about the position of the head on the vertebral column, and its "primary control" (to the student of animal behaviour, who notices that the head, as the bearer of the long-distance sense organs, usually initiates change of movements of the whole body, it sounds highly plausible that the head-neck region should have a certain dominance in the control of posture and body movement). From the study of fossils of our ancestors it is clear that there is a consistent trend in the evolution of the position of the head. What has happened is this: in our early ancestors the head (with a smaller brain than ours and larger jaws) was not precisely balanced on the vertebral column. The centre of gravity of their heads was situated well forward of the points at which the skull rests on the vertebral column, the condyli. As "humanization" proceeded, the centre of gravity of the skull moved nearer a position above the condyli. However, even in modern Man the condyli lie somewhat behind the head's centre of gravity. From these peculiarities of the head-neck region of successive stages in the hominid line it has been concluded that this region has only gradually adapted to the upright body position. This sounds plausible enough. But the additional implications have been made that (1) our early ancestors, with their more forward placed heads, had less good use than we; and (2) that (because even we are not fully aligned) our evolution towards uprightness and bipedalism has not yet been completed. For various reasons I do not believe in these further implications. Firstly, as far as we can see, all animals (apart from excessively domesticated and some zoo animals) have, in Alexander terms, good, even excellent use, i.e. their movements and the skeleto-muscular apparatus function very efficiently. Second, as we have seen, our forebears began to evolve bipedalism at least five million years ago; this long period should be more than sufficient to develop the upright stance to maximum efficiency; if our head-neck region is not precisely aligned in the above sense, it must be for other reasons. Thirdly, when we say that our remote ancestors must have had bad use because they held their heads further forward than we do, we forget that they had a different build than we. It is of course build and movement together ("functioning structures") that determine efficiency. What we *can* say is that if one of *us* would walk with his head so far forward he would use himself badly. How unjustified it is in principle to pronounce about the alleged use of, say, *Homo erectus*, or Neanderthal Man becomes clear when we carry this argument *ad absurdum* and say that a dog, and even more so a rhino, must have bad use because they carry their heads so far in front of their bodies. Fourthly, we have very clear evidence of the almost unbelievable toughness and hunting abilities of these early men. Where in the modern world would we find men who, with the very primitive weapons at their disposal, could overpower mammoths and other elephants, woolly rhinoceroses, and horses? In order to live the way they did, they must surely have had *better* use than any of us! Fifthly, there are even now relic populations of hunter-gatherers who, though contemporaries of us, have retained a way of life very similar to that of our (and their) ancestors. They all belong to the modern species *Homo sapiens*, but are genetically different sub-species or sub-sub-species. It is believed that of all these ethnic groups, such as the Bushmen, the Pigmies, the Australian Aborigines and the Eskimo, the Bushmen have deviated least from the life style of our pre-agricultural ancestors. They have been studied just in time, and some of their hunting expeditions have even been filmed. We can draw more than one lesson from the evidence. Firstly, they are undoubtedly genetically different from us, and this expresses itself in their use: one of their striking traits is a pronounced lordosis. If a modern Caucasian ("white man") were to come to an Alexander teacher with this degree of lordosis, his teacher would (rightly) want to work on this deviation. When Bushmen sit, they bend their backs in a way that an Alexander teacher would abhor. In Bushmen, however, both postures are normal, and, as all observers agree, they have magnificent use, at the same time efficient and graceful. This emphasizes once again that, just as with our remote ancestors, use must be considered in relation to build. The other interesting point about the Bushmen is that they too are extremely tough and efficient hunters. How efficient they are is also indicated by the fact that even those who live in semi-deserts spend on average no more than sixteen hours a week on collecting food!

Before returning to my original question a few words must be said about an aspect of our evolution that has no equivalent in the animal world.

The Cultural evolution
The invasion of a new niche is in evolution nothing special; throughout the past numerous new forms have branched off by this very same process. What makes the human case unique is that his ecological switch occurred at a time and a phase in the history of the mammals when a number of "predispositions" had developed, such as the use of arms and hands for swinging, leaving the legs available

for walking; "small-group sociality"; and of course a considerable capacity of the brain, unique even among the primates.

Apart from enabling us to enter the rich but dangerous niche of the plains, our brain has also been responsible for something that is literally without precedent. Superimposed on the, still on-going, genetic evolution a fundamentally new type of evolution has emerged. A considerable time ago—certainly more than 100,000 years—we have begun to transfer, from generation to generation, not only genetic instructions, but also individually acquired knowledge. Such "cultural" transfer can occur occasionally and on a modest scale in some animals, but in the human species it has become the main source of change. Each generation adds new experience and even inventions to what it has learned from its elders, and so the transfer becomes cumulative, and also, inevitably, accelerating. The genome keeps evolving in its own slow way, but the cultural evolution, initially without doubt also slow, has since long outpaced genetic change. The early, slow but soon accelerating growth of cultural progress can be seen very clearly for instance in the progress of the flint-working skill since over a million years ago. An elegant way of demonstrating this is to measure the total length of cutting edge of all pieces obtained by working, say, one pound of solid flint. At first slowly, then faster and faster, this cutting edge length increases, until a stage is reached at which, after trimming, to start with a flint nodule into a regular cylinder, the entire block is cut up into elegant, knife-shaped sherds. Such a magnificent skill can only be transferred culturally.

Since the stone ages the cultural evolution has of course come very much further; and has in fact accelerated in an almost breath-taking way. Change has become so explosive that all of us become Rip van Winkles within our lifetime.

For my present purpose two aspects of the cultural evolution are of special interest. Firstly, medical and other technologies have reduced early mortality, so that many more offspring reach maturity than are required for replacement; this has led to the "population explosion". Apart from its deadly overall dangers, such as famine, this population growth has also led to greatly increased local densities, particularly in cities and megalopolises. Secondly, and even more important, we have, rather than maintaining ourselves in our habitat, literally conquered it, and increasingly changed it. Both socially and physically we live in a world very different from that which genetic evolution has adapted us to. Admittedly, many aspects of our new environment are life enhancing, and to that extent cultural evolution is (as it was intended to be from the start) part of the adaptation process. But many of the new changes have turned out to be harmful; we need only to think of the effects on the human population of over-exploitation of resources; of our failure to provide everyone with sufficient food; of hundreds of kinds of pollution—physical, bio-logical, and social. I shall not here dwell on the calamitous nature of these trends in the present stage of our evolution but will now return to our original question.

The Origin of Misuse

As remarked earlier, we can discern, in the Alexander literature, two notions about the genesis of misuse and about what Alexandering does. I believe that, although these views are not incompatible and each of them may be partly true, it is important to distinguish them sharply as concepts. As mentioned before, one is that we are still on our way to the evolution of a more erect posture, and that Alexan-dering anticipates and works ahead towards our future genetic evolution. I have argued why I feel that this view is not supported by the facts, but springs from the mistaken idea that our ancestors of, for example, the *erectus* and Neanderthal stages must have had bad use. Of course we have not seen them move, but we do have an abundance of fossil evidence of their prowess and toughness. Nor does our present, "imperfect" alignment of the centre of gravity of our heads and our condyli necessarily mean that we shall evolve further in the direction of perfect alignment. We just can't predict what will happen in the distant future, and for all we know the present condition may well be, for us, the best possible compromise between a number of different demands. I do not think that the peculiarities of our head-neck region have been studied from this point of view. Seeing that our upright posture has a history of at least five million years, it would seem most likely that every stage of the pre-human and the human line has had, for its purpose, good use. I submit therefore (without altogether excluding the possibility) that there simply is no evidence in favour of the idea that our head-neck region is "not yet there" and that Alexandering pushes us forward to a future ideal.

The second idea, that bad use is a recent, environment-induced, degenerative phenomenon, has much more in its favour than could have been realized 50, even 20 years ago. There are quite a number of indications that our modern, man-made environment is now exerting new pressures which overstretch our adjustability. First of all, and already well known in Alexander's time: the members of modern, urban, industrialized society simply sit far too much and walk far too little. Misuse of our bodies of this kind has started very long ago, in fact as soon as division of labour began. There are suggestions that already the late stone ages have produced specialized flint workers, who may well have spent far more time at their craft than at food-getting. Up to a point this switch to more sitting could be supposed to have done little harm, but in our affluent societies the last one, two, and here and there three generations have become almost totally sessile. Schools were bad enough long before any of us was born, but while now at least primary schools allow for a little more mobility, cars and television have more than undone this little improvement; some years ago it was reported that the average American spends over 24 hours a week sitting in front of the television set.

Much less attention has been given in Alexander circles (and in medicine) to our present food situation. Two aspects deserve mention. Firstly, people in affluent societies simply eat too much. I feel that it is worth investigating whether the undeniable, non-genetic increase in tallness that we have witnessed in this century at least in affluent societies can have to do with this overfeeding and/or with changes in the composition of our food. This tallness, together with flabbiness of the under-used muscles, cannot but put a severe strain on the musculature of the vertebral column. Secondly, the composition of our food has changed drastically in recent times. Many of these changes are not visible, nor do even appeal to our tastes. On the one hand much of our food is now short of a number of vitamins and some minerals, and vitamin deficiencies, including even scurvy, are making their appearance again. At the same time we are fed willy nilly numerous additives, some of which are harmful. There is a growing nutritional literature, which reports on these cultural changes in our food, and remedial action may well become possible, though undoubtedly not in the near future.

Finally, much misuse is a form of response to psychological pressures. Many parts of our bodies are employed in a rich repertoire of movements called the "expressions of the emotions". Perhaps the most relevant example is the "cowed" posture, in which the shoulders are held up and forward and the neck is drawn in downward. Its most pronounced form, usually taken up for a moment only, is the "startle response". The less extreme cowed posture is normally adopted for somewhat longer but still limited times. But very many people in modern society "freeze" in this position and maintain it, often for hours on end, during walking, standing, and other activities. In many it has become *the* habitual posture. The freezing phenomenon can also be seen in such seemingly trivial and restricted movements as the brief raising of the eyebrows and simultaneous lifting of the skin of the forehead that people do (in many cultures) when addressed by, or addressing someone else in a friendly, interested way. There are people who, when involved in an interesting discussion, keep their eyebrows up throughout the interaction. Others have a permanent frown, will continuously gnash their teeth, keep their jaws locked, etc. These minor movements are not unimportant because, as every Alexander teacher knows, and I think most pupils have experienced, they go together with numerous forms of muscular tension elsewhere in the body. Movements and gestures that "express the emotions" are almost invariably due to ambivalent emotional tension, and I am convinced that their perpetuation in a "frozen" state reveals abnormally high tension, and that this is a condition conducive to the development of misuse.

When we now try to weigh the various arguments for and against the two hypotheses about the origin of misuse—that of "unfinished" genetic evolution and that of phenotypic deterioration in response to a changed environment—it will be clear that, for the reasons given, I feel that the first interpretation has little to recommend it, whereas that of misuse as a "civilization-illness" is supported by quite suggestive evidence. Accordingly, I think that we must definitely view the Alexander Technique as a re-education rather than as a form of "further education", i.e. of mimicking what we expect will be our future genetic evolution.

If this view of misuse as a non-genetic modification is correct, it is easier to understand why Alexandering is in many cases so effective, for individually acquired deviations are as a rule more amenable to treatment than are genetic defects. On the other hand, this environmental, "experiential" interpretation of misuse makes us at the same time expect that it will become both more pronounced and more widespread in the not too distant future. No generation has been exposed to such a degree to the pressures mentioned as the one that is now growing up, and its members may therefore well develop, in ten or twenty years' time, more pronounced "Alexanderable" symptoms than our generation.

How will the future cope with this expected increase in numbers of persons in need of Alexandering? If misuse is indeed, and will increasingly become, such a general phenomenon, it will of course be impossible to provide for Alexander lessons for all those in need, even if the medical profession and the physiotherapists were to become more convinced of the value of the technique. It may therefore be necessary to consider possibilities for prevention. This too will not be easy. Again, if our environment and our pathological response to it are to blame, we would have to aim at the same time at making our environment less damaging, and at bolstering people's resistance. However, most of the pressures I mentioned (those related to eating, sitting, psychological stress) are so inherent in the progress of our civilization that they will not easily be changed. Even so, since my interpretation is both tentative and vague, further research into the problem will have to decide what are the main stresses involved, and what counter measures are needed and possible. And this leads us to the realization that the problem of misuse may well be a part of the much wider issue of stress diseases. The note on which I end is therefore too familiar: before effective prevention will be possible, the causes of misuse will have to be much better understood, and this will require time-consuming and costly research.

But if a reduction of the pressures exerted by the modern environment seems to be unlikely at least for the time being, the resilience of those who have to live in it and to cope with it can obviously be restored to quite an extent, and it seems clear that the Alexander Technique can play its part here too—that it can be preventive as well as curing.

From what I have said it will be obvious that, once I began to pay attention to the problem of the origin of misuse, I became even more convinced than I had been on purely empirical grounds, not only of the great potential of the Alexander Technique, but also of its biological soundness and plausibility. We must hope that an increasing number of those who are suffering from misuse will come to share this conviction and give the technique a try.

TWENTY-EIGHT

Alexander's Meeting with Coghill
by Edward H. Owen

F.M. ALEXANDER'S meeting in America in 1940 with the American naturalist, George Ellett Coghill, was an occasion that was followed with keen interest by the small circle that knew something of both men's work.

Here were two dedicated investigators—both, in Professor Coghill's words, "technically laymen so far as the medical profession is concerned"—who for many years had been independently exploring the field of functioning in relation to the total pattern of the organism. Their approaches were very different, Coghill studying the problem through the structure and development of the lower vertebrates, Alexander in the re-education of human beings; but those who had had an opportunity to compare their results were convinced that many of their observations and conclusions were strikingly in accord. As early as 1937, Dr Peter Macdonald wrote to the *British Medical Journal* pointing out that Coghill's anatomical work on the large American type of newt, Amblystoma, provided scientific confirmation of Alexander's discovery of the "primary control". In the world of biology, Coghill was—as A. Rugg-Gunn put it—"the first to emphasize the primacy of the total pattern and, as a corollary, the secondary character of local reflexes".

It was the American journalist, Arthur F. Busch, who first brought Coghill and Alexander into personal touch. In an article on Coghill in the 7 April 1939, issue of *The Brooklyn Citizen*, Busch—writing under his pen-name of Michael March—drew attention to the fact that "Mr Alexander's technique for the restoration of the total integration of the individual approaches the individual as an integrated whole", and declared that "Professor Coghill's findings confirm the scientific basis of Alexander's practical work". This article led to correspondence between Coghill, Busch and Alexander, and to Alexander sending the American naturalist copies of *Man's Supreme Inheritance* and *Constructive Conscious Control*.

In a letter to Alexander of 4 June 1939, acknowledging the books, Coghill wrote: "I am reading these with a great deal of interest and profit, amazed to see how you, years ago, discovered in human physiology and psychology the same principles which I worked out in

the behaviour of lower vertebrates." Alexander had offered to give
Coghill a practical demonstration of his teaching if he could manage
to come to London. To this the other replied: "I am very restricted
in my activities by a bad heart and numerous complications . . . I
have been practically in this condition, fluctuating between hope and
despair, for five years. I must be near the end of my career. I can
scarcely hope to go to London as I would like to do." That was
shortly before the outbreak of war. It seemed equally unlikely at that
time that Alexander, by then in his 70s, would be visiting America
again, although during the 1920s he had had a flourishing teaching
practice there. His brother, A. R. Alexander, had settled in the States
to carry on the work. When war broke out, however, a number of
Alexander's supporters—among them Stafford Cripps—felt it was
imperative that, as the founder of a teaching method that might be
lost to mankind for good, Alexander should remove himself and one
or two of his assistant teachers from the immediate threat of bombing
and invasion. In July 1940, therefore, Alexander, together with Ethel
Webb, Margaret Goldie, Irene Stewart and a number of children
from their "little school" at Penhill in Kent, were evacuated to
America, where they were accommodated in the famous Whitney
Homestead at Stowe, Massachusetts.

Unexpectedly, a meeting between Coghill and Alexander had
now become practicable. The American naturalist, weakened by
his recurrent heart attacks but still struggling to continue his
research work, was living with his daughter Muriel on a property
he had named "The Singing Pines", at Gainesville, Florida. As
soon as there was an opportunity, Alexander went south to see
him.

The meeting was marked by mutual liking and respect. Alexander
wrote later in a letter to Coghill's friend, collaborator and biographer,
Professor C. Judson Herrick: "My meeting with Coghill was a notable
and valuable happening in my 81 years' experience." Coghill himself
wrote to a friend: "Mr Alexander seems to me to be a very unusual
man. He has grasped the same scientific principles through practical
work with human beings that I have found through my investigations
of detailed anatomy in the lower forms."

A warm friendship was struck up—though a brief one, for Coghill
had not many more months of life before him. There were few
visitors to "The Singing Pines", and undoubtedly it cheered the sick
man to be able to talk to someone about the progress of his work—
and to unburden himself of some of the sense of injustice and frustration he felt as a result of his dismissal in later life from the staff of the

Wistar Institute of Anatomy and Biology, where he had worked for ten years.

Alexander gave Coghill many hours of teaching during that weekend in an effort to relieve the condition that was making any exertion increasingly difficult for him. The experience of having Alexander's hands on him proved an exciting revelation to Coghill. As the lesson proceeded, he explained to his daughter: "It's the growth process!"—the process that his researches had convinced him must be present in all living organisms and which he now found explicitly recognized and employed in Alexander's teaching technique. He agreed to write a foreword to *The Universal Constant in Living*, which Alexander had completed during a three months' holiday in Maine and which was due to be published later that year. Here he stated:

Mr Alexander has demonstrated the very important psychological principle that the proprioceptive system can be brought under conscious control, and can be educated to carry to the motor centres the stimulus which is responsible for the muscular activity which brings about the manner of working [use] of the mechanism . . . I regard his methods as thoroughly scientific and educationally sound.

Alexander was saddened by the physical condition of his new friend and by his personal difficulties. On his return to New York he did his best to use his influence to gain some redress for Coghill, but without success.

The last contact between them was within a few weeks of Coghill's death in July 1941. Alexander had written inviting him to come and stay at the Whitney Homestead and Coghill had accepted. Then came the news from Muriel Coghill that her father had had a relapse. From this final attack he never recovered.

C. Judson Herrick has written of Coghill that he was "a naturalist in the proper meaning of that term, a student of nature, thorough-going and uncompromising, not a mere bug-hunter or pebble-picker. All his thinking was naturalistic. . . . His philosophic interests developed in a natural way, directly out of his own experiences as an acute observer of the vital processes and the organs involved." These words could well apply, too, to the fellow "layman" whose visit meant so much to Coghill in his last months.

TWENTY-NINE

The Total Pattern of Behaviour
by Dr Wilfred Barlow

F. M. ALEXANDER and Professor G. E. Coghill came into contact relatively late in life, during world war II, when Alexander had been evacuated with his school to America. There had been a certain amount of prior correspondence, in which Coghill had written: "I am amazed to see how you, years ago, discovered in human physiology and psychology the same principle which I worked out in the behaviour of lower vertebrates."

Coghill was one of the earliest neuropsychiatrists: that is to say, he was a neurologist who tried to link up his subject with psychology. In his own words, he "became aware that the natural approach to the kind of psychological information he wanted lay through the physiology of the nervous system". The organism upon which he carried out most of his research was a primitive vertebrate, the axolotl (a type of newt), and he described his experiments in his book, *Anatomy and the Problem of Behaviour*, published in 1929. The purpose of his experiments on the growing axolotl was to observe the manner in which it began to move as its neuromuscular system developed, and to correlate these movements with an anatomical study of its nervous system. He carried out the study throughout the early movements of swimming, up to the moment when it learned to walk on land. In these observations, he found that the pattern of movements is "cephalocaudal", that is to say, it starts at the head and proceeds tailwards: the musculature at the head end is the first part to contract in response to any stimulus, and the wave of neuromuscular activity then proceeds tailwards. In Alexander terms, "the head leads and the body follows". The movement of the limbs in the early stages is always bound up with the trunk reaction: the limbs do not move unless the trunk moves first. Coghill termed this primary dominance of the trunk over the limbs the "total pattern of reaction", in contradistinction to "partial patterns of reaction" which later develop in the limbs as they acquire partial independence.

This work on "total pattern" and "partial pattern" was welcomed by many psychologists of the Gestalt school. If I understand it rightly, the Gestalt school stands for total unity as the dominant principle governing mental processes; pure simple sensations, they say, do not exist as such, but the apparently particular elements in consciousness emerge from a general field and exist only in relation to that field. They are concerned with the "whole man" or the "organism as a whole", so they not unnaturally took up gladly this work of Coghill's, undeterred by the popular expression "To be as inebriated as a newt", which might seem to imply a certain lack of wholeness.

The Total Pattern of Integration

Coghill's studies were also extremely welcome to Alexander, and in his later years Alexander adapted his concept of a "primary control" —in which the head leads and the body follows—to suggest that it was based on Coghill's "total pattern" mechanism for the integration of posture and movement. Alexander's point was that this mechanism, which should work automatically from its position in the mid-brain (the "old brain"), may be interfered with by conscious impulses which are being sent down from the "new brain", that is to say, the cerebral cortex. He suggested that the majority of human beings, under the influence of urban civilization, react habitually in such a way as to interfere with this integrating mechanism in the mid-brain. The "total pattern of reaction", which should be maintained by the dominance of the head-neck relationship, becomes sacrificed in the hurry and flurry of modern life, to "partial patterns of reaction" in the limbs: for example, the pianist, who is concerned especially with movements of his hands, may disregard the need to maintain the integrity of the vertebral pattern: but equally, the housewife at the sink, or the car driver at the wheel, may lose such total pattern dominance.

Psychosomatic Conflict

Coghill himself saw clearly the connection between Alexander's re-educational approach and his own description of the imbalance which may arise between the total pattern and partial patterns.

That this is more than theory Mr Alexander demonstrated to me in lessons which he kindly gave me. He enabled me to prevent misdirection of the muscles of my neck and back, and to bring about a use of these muscles that determined the relative position of my head and neck to my body and so on to my limbs. This led to changes in the muscular and other conditions throughout my body and limbs associated with a pattern of behaviour more in agreement with the total pattern. The whole procedure was calculated to occupy my brain with the projection of directive messages that would enable me to acquire conscious control of the proprioceptive component of the reflex mechanism involved. It is my opinion that habitual use of improper reflex mechanisms in sitting, standing and walking introduces conflict in the nervous system, and that this conflict is the cause of fatigue and nervous strain, which brings many ills in their train. Mr Alexander, by relieving this conflict between the total pattern which is hereditary and innate, and reflex mechanisms which are individually cultivated, conserves the energies of the nervous system, and by so doing corrects not only the postural difficulties but also many other pathological conditions that are not ordinarily recognized as postural. The variable and relative dominance of the organism-as-a-whole over its parts is the key to psychosomatic medicine. The relationship is real and physiological, not imaginary and vitalistic or spiritualistic. . . . The extreme defect in the organism-as-a-whole occurs in split personality or in multiple personality. Here the whole overt behaviour pattern passes under the dominance of an individuated sector of the organism-as-a-whole, which introspectively seems to the individual consciousness like another person. Probably all mental conflict may be similarly explained.

Tinbergen's Views on Coghill

In retrospect, it appears that Alexander's supporters, myself included, overemphasized the possibility that Coghill had given good scientific backing for his ideas. In recent years, it has seemed more and more likely that a large part of Alexander-learning is by the addition of separately learned components, rather than simply by differentiation out of a generalized total pattern. When I wrote to Professor Tinbergen to this effect, asking for permission to publish a section which he had written on Coghill in his *Study of Instinct*, he was glad to give permission. His reply to me is a useful introduction to this extract.

By all means do quote the Coghill passage from *The Study of Instinct*. Although the book is now grossly outdated, this particular section has lost nothing of its basic correctness. It is one of those examples where an author has written something on rather intuitive grounds, which later work has confirmed. I have now an idea (although I could not possibly write a comprehensive treatise on it) that Coghill's views are valid for the kind of early, low-level movement-systems that he investigated, e.g. the earliest phases of co-ordinated locomotion. Later on in the development, integrative, "constructive" processes may be the rule. For example, complex feeding behaviour chains in some birds appear first as disconnected components (1) in any sequence, (2) aimed at any type of object, and (3) with poor co-ordination and orientation. Partly through internal maturation, but largely through the contribution made by various learning processes, these three types of imperfections are corrected. So rather than differentiation with time, such cases show integration or construction with time, and this may well be the rule where learning is involved. The whole story of behaviour ontogeny has now shown itself to be incredibly complex, but I am sure that these *two* principles are valid, and I am pretty confident that Coghill's type applies to early and simple systems. I can imagine that, as you say, the Alexander training "uses" the second strategy, but I feel I cannot judge that because I do not yet see the interplay between this "additive" learning and the unmistakable fact that every pupil has, already from long before the start of a course of Alexander lessons, an integrated, web-like system of movements (however ill-performed).

Extract from The Study of Instinct *by Professor N. Tinbergen*
A parallel study of developmental processes in the nervous system and in behaviour has been carried out by Coghill (1929) for the early stages of behaviour in the axolotl larva. Coghill observed that the earliest appearance of certain movements occurred simultaneously with the appearance of certain nervous connections which, by their topography, were thought to mediate these movements. Thus, the first movement is a reflex flexure of the anterior trunk muscles opposite to the stimulated side. With increasing age, the area of muscle involved extends farther tailward, until at last the whole trunk responds by "coiling". Now at the time when the first flexure movement was performed, neurological examination detected the first cross-connection between the sensory and the motor paths, the so-called floor cells. The gradual tailward extension of the flexure coincides with a spreading of the development of the motor cells from the front, where development begins, to the rear.

At the next stage the body can be bent into an "S". At this stage a coil begins in the anterior region and spreads tailward, but before the contraction has reached the tail, a new, reversed flexure appears at the head. The appearance of this "S" flexure coincides with the development of connections between the sensory cells and the motor cells of the same side.

Although Coghill's interpretation of the swimming rhythm is based on the chain reflex scheme, which is now considered an incomplete and, in a way, inadequate picture, his observations must, of course, be accepted and they show that nerve growth and development of behaviour go hand in hand.

It is not necessary to elaborate this point further; we may safely assume that development of overt behaviour usually is the result of growth processes in the nervous system and not growth of muscles or receptor organs, which, as a general rule, are developed earlier. So far as is known, only the very earliest movements of developing embryos are usually myogenic. . . .

As I have mentioned, the movements in the first stages of development are simultaneous, mass movements of the trunk somites. The general course of further development is that the mass movements differentiate into patterns, the components of which gradually become distinct from the behaviour as a whole. A differentiated pattern of locomotion does not arise by construction, by addition of parts, but in just the reverse way, by differentiation of a diffuse whole. For instance, the limbs in Amblystoma at first are only capable of moving synchronously with, and in the same way as, the neighbouring trunk somites. Later they are able to move relatively independently. In a comparable way, gill movements are at first completely dependent on trunk movements; they become capable of independent movements later on.

The differentiation of feeding behaviour follows another course. The complete feeding behaviour of the larva consists of a forward leap, accompanied by snapping and subsequent swallowing. The order of appearance is: first the leap is shown alone, later actual snapping is added, while swallowing is added later still. This type of development *could properly be called addition rather than differentiation.*

Although there are many scattered reports about the appearance of certain reactions as a whole—such as feeding, escape, etc.—analyses of such movements together with a study of the incipient stages such as that presented by Coghill are seldom given. From what we know of the order of appearance of reactions, it appears that each species has a fixed time pattern just as with growing morphological structures. A fine instance of study of such a time pattern is Mrs Nice's work on the development of behaviour of the song sparrow.

As an instance of analytical work in this field, the thorough study made by Kortlandt of the European cormorant may be cited. Kortlandt studied the ontogenic development of several behaviour patterns, and found, contrary to what we could expect from a generalization of Coghill's results on the locomotion pattern, that the *component parts mature independently and are later combined into purposive patterns of a higher order*. Thus complete nesting behaviour consists of fetching twigs, pushing them into the nest, and fastening them there by the typical quivering movement shown by so many birds. The young begin to show nesting behaviour at an age of two weeks. This consists merely of quivering, which is performed quite "senselessly", for the twigs are not fastened. When four or five weeks old, the young continue quivering until the twig gets caught by the nest. Still later they accept twigs from the male and also go to fetch twigs for themselves to work them into the nest.

Our analysis of instinctive behaviour allows us to describe this in more general terms: the lower units, at the level of the consummatory acts, appear first and the appetitive behaviour appears later.

A similar process seems to occur in the development of the pattern of feeding the young. The complete pattern consists of regurgitating and then opening the mouth, bending over the young and then allowing it to put its head into the mouth. Young of two-and-a-half to three weeks of age show the first incipient feeding behaviour without the introductory regurgitating. Here again the consummatory act appears first and the introductory behaviour follows much later.

It would seem to me that no general descriptive rules of the onto-genetic development of instinctive behaviour can be established until we know a good deal more. It would be of special importance to give attention not only to the appearance of individual components but also to the development of pattern in relation to that of its component parts. *It seems that one cannot generalize Coghill's con-clusion that individual acts of behaviour "crystallize out" from a diffuse total response*, and that a kind of *additive* type of integration may play a part too, perhaps especially in the higher levels. In this respect it is certainly of considerable interest that the development of Amblystoma's feeding reaction, being a response of a higher level than the locomotion responses, seems to follow a course more similar to that described by Kortlandt than to that found by Coghill for locomotion.

APPLICATIONS

MEDICAL

THIRTY

Ethology and Stress Diseases
by N. Tinbergen, F.R.S.

(This article is the oration Professor Tinbergen delivered in Stockholm on 12 December 1973 when he received the Nobel Prize for Physiology or Medicine, a prize he shared with K. Lorenz and K. von Frisch. Minor corrections and additions have been made by the author.)

MANY OF US have been surprised at the unconventional decision of the Nobel Foundation to award this year's prize for Physiology or Medicine to three men who had until recently been regarded as "mere animal watchers". Since at least Konrad Lorenz and I could not really be described as physiologists, we must conclude that our *scientia amabilis* is now being acknowledged as an integral part of the eminently practical field of medicine. It is for this reason that I have decided to discuss today two concrete examples of how the old method[1] of "watching and wondering" about behaviour (which incidentally we reviewed rather than invented) can indeed contribute to the relief of human suffering, in particular of suffering caused by stress. It seems to me fitting to do this in a city already renowned for important work on psychosocial stress and psychosomatic diseases.[2]

[The first part of the article then dealt with Professor Tinbergen's research into early childhood Autism, which is not reprinted here.]

. . . My second example of the usefulness of an ethological approach to medicine has quite a different history. It concerns the work of a very remarkable man, the late F. M. Alexander.[3] His research started some 50 years before the revival of ethology, for which we are now being honoured, yet his procedure was very similar to modern observational methods, and we believe that his achievements and those of his pupils deserve close attention.

Alexander, who was born in 1869 in Tasmania, became at an early age a "reciter of dramatic and humorous pieces". Very soon he developed serious vocal trouble and he came very near to losing his voice altogether. When no doctor could help him, he took matters into his own hands. He began to observe himself in front of a mirror, and then he noticed that his voice was at its worst when he adopted the stances which to him felt appropriate and right for what he was reciting. Without any outside help he worked out, during a series of agonizing years, how to improve what is now called the "use" of his body musculature in all his postures and movements. And, the remarkable outcome was that he regained control of his voice. This story, of perceptiveness, of intelligence, and of persistence, shown by a man without medical training, is one of the true epics of medical research and practice.[4]

Once Alexander had become aware of the misuse of his own body, he began to observe his fellow men, and he found that, at least in modern western society, the majority of people stand, sit, and move in an equally defective manner.

Encouraged by a doctor in Sydney, he now became a kind of missionary. He set out to teach—first actors, then a variety of people —how to restore the proper use of their musculature. Gradually he discovered that he could in this way alleviate an astonishing variety of somatic and mental illnesses. He also wrote extensively on the subject. And finally he taught a number of his pupils to become teachers in their turn, and to achieve the same results with their patients. Whereas it had taken him years to work out the technique and to apply it to his own body, a successful course became a matter of months, with occasional refresher sessions afterwards. Admittedly, the training of a good Alexander teacher takes a few years.

For scores of years a small but dedicated number of pupils have continued his work. Their combined successes have recently been described by Barlow.[5] I must admit that his physiological explanations of how the treatment could be supposed to work (and also a touch of hero worship in his book) made me initially a little doubtful and even sceptical. But the claims made, first by Alexander, and reiterated and extended by Barlow, sounded so extraordinary that I felt I ought to give the method at least the benefit of the doubt. And so, arguing that medical practice often goes by the sound empirical principle of "the proof of the pudding is in the eating", my wife, one of our daughters, and I decided to undergo treatment ourselves, and also to use the opportunity for observing its effects as critically as we could. For obvious reasons, each of use went to a different Alexander teacher.

We discovered that the therapy is based on exceptionally sophisticated observation, not only by means of vision but also to a surprising extent by using the sense of touch. It consists in essence of no more than a very gentle, first exploratory, and then corrective manipulation of the entire muscular system. This starts with the head and neck, then very soon the shoulders and chest are involved, and finally the pelvis, legs, and feet, until the whole body is under scrutiny and treatment. As in our own observations of children, the therapist is continuously monitoring the body, and adjusting his procedure all the time. What is actually done varies from one patient to another, depending on what kind of misuse the diagnostic exploration reveals. And naturally, it affects different people in different ways. But between the three of us, we already notice, with growing amazement,

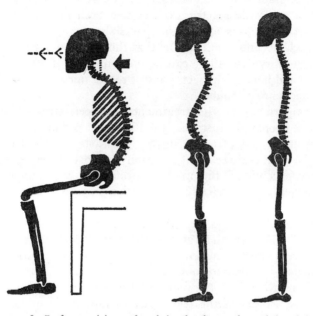

Figure 8. Left: position of pelvis, back, neck and head in slumping position (compare Plate 12). Centre: standing in hunched position. Right: well balanced.

very striking improvements in such diverse things as high blood pressure, breathing, depth of sleep, overall cheerfulness and mental alertness, resilience against outside pressures, and also in such a refined skill as playing a stringed instrument.

So from personal experience we can already confirm some of the seemingly fantastic claims made by Alexander and his followers, namely, that many types of underperformance and even ailments, both mental and physical, can be alleviated, sometimes to a surprising extent, by teaching the body musculature to function differently. And although we have by no means finished our course, the evidence given and documented by Alexander and Barlow of beneficial effects on a variety of vital functions no longer sounds so astonishing to us. Their long list includes first of all what Barlow calls the "rag bag" of rheumatism, including various forms of arthritis, then respiratory troubles, and even potentially lethal asthma; following in their wake, circulation defects, which may lead to high blood pressure and also to some dangerous heart conditions; gastrointestinal disorders of many types; various gynaecological conditions; sexual failures; migraines and depressive states that often lead to suicide; in short, a very wide spectrum of diseases, both somatic and mental, that are not caused by identifiable parasites.

Although no one would claim that the Alexander treatment is a cure-all in every case, there can be no doubt that if often does have profound and beneficial effects; and, I repeat once more, both in the mental and somatic sphere.

The importance of the treatment has been stressed by many prominent people, for instance, John Dewey,[6] Aldous Huxley,[7] and, perhaps more convincing to us, by scientists of renown, such as Coghill,[8] Dart,[9] and the great neurophysiologist Sherrington.[10] Yet, with few exceptions, the medical profession has largely ignored Alexander, perhaps under the impression that he was the centre of some kind of cult, and also because the effects seemed difficult to explain. And this brings me to my next point.

Once one knows that an empirically developed therapy has demonstrable effects, one likes to know how it could work—what its physiological explanation could be. And here some recent discoveries in the borderline field between neurophysiology and ethology can make some aspects of the Alexander therapy more understandable and more plausible than they could have been in Sherrington's time.

One of these new discoveries concerns the key concept of reafference.[11] There are many strong indications that, at various levels of integration, from single muscle units up to complex behaviour, the correct performance of many movements is continuously checked by the brain. It does this by comparing a feedback report that says "orders carried out" with the feedback expectation for which, with the initiation of each movement, the brain has been altered. Only when the expected feedback and the actual feedback match does the brain stop sending out commands for corrective action. Already the discoverers of this principle, von Holst and Mittelstaedt, knew that the functioning of this complex mechanism could vary from moment to moment with the internal state of the subject—the "target value" or *Sollwert* of the expected feedback changes with the motor commands that are given. But what Alexander has discovered beyond this is that a lifelong misuse of the body muscles (such as caused by, for instance, too much sitting and too little walking) can make the entire system go wrong. As a consequence, reports that "all is correct" are received by the brain (or perhaps interpreted as correct) when in fact all is very wrong. A person can feel at ease, for example, when slouching in front of a television set, when in fact he is grossly abusing his body. I can show you only a few examples, but they will be familiar to all of you (plates 12 to 15, taken from *The Alexander Principle*).

It is still an open question exactly where in this complex mechanism the matching procedure goes wrong under the influence of consistent misuse. But the modern ethologist feels inclined, with Alexander and Barlow, to blame phenotypic rather than genetic causes for misuse. It is highly unlikely that in their very long evolutionary history of walking upright, the hominids have not had time to evolve the correct mechanisms for bipedal locomotion. This conclusion receives support from the surprising, but indubitable fact that even after 40 to 50 years of obvious misuse one's body can (one might say) snap back into proper, and in many respects more healthy, use as a result of a short series of half-hourly sessions. Proper stance and movement are obviously genetically old, environment-resistant behaviours.[12] Misuse, with all its psychosomatic, or rather somatopsychic, consequences must therefore be considered a result of modern living conditions of a culturally determined stress. I might add here that I am not merely thinking of too much sitting, but just as much of the cowed posture that one assumes when one feels that one is not quite up to one's work, when one feels insecure.

Second, it need not cause surprise that a mere gentle handling of body muscles can have such profound effects on both body and mind. The more that is being discovered about psychosomatic diseases, and in general about the extremely complex two-way traffic between the brain and the rest of the body, the more obvious it has become that too rigid a distinction between mind and body is of only limited use to medical science, in fact can be a hindrance to its advance.

A third biologically interesting aspect of the Alexander therapy is that every session clearly demonstrates that the innumerable muscles of the body are continuously operating as an intricately linked web. Whenever a gentle pressure is used to make a slight change in leg posture, the neck muscles react immediately. Conversely, when the therapist helps one to release the neck muscles, it is amazing to see quite pronounced movements, for instance of the toes, even when one is lying on a couch.

In this short sketch, I can do no more than characterize, and recommend, the Alexander treatment as an extremely sophisticated form of rehabilitation, or rather of redeployment, of the entire muscular equipment, and through that of many other organs. Compared with this, many types of physiotherapy which are now in general use look surprisingly crude and restricted in their effect, and sometimes even harmful to the rest of the body.

What then is the upshot of these few brief remarks about the Alexander treatment? First of all they stress the importance for medical science of open-minded observation—of "watching and wondering". This basic scientific method is still too often looked down on by those blinded by the glamour of apparatus, by the prestige of tests, and by the temptation to turn to drugs. But it is by using this old method of observation that the general misuse of the body can be seen in a new light; to a much larger extent than is now realized it could very well be due to modern stressful conditions.

But beyond this I feel that my excursion into the field of medical research has much wider implications. Medical science and practice meet with a growing sense of unease and of lack of confidence from the side of the general public. The causes of this are complex, but at least in one respect the situation could be improved: a little more open-mindedness, a little more collaboration with other biological sciences, and a little more attention to the body as a whole and to the unity of body and mind could substantially enrich the field of medical research. I therefore appeal to our medical colleagues to recognize that the study of animals—in particular "plain" observation—can make useful contributions to human biology not only in the field of somatic malfunctioning, but also in that of behavioural disturbances, and ultimately help us to understand what psychosocial stress is doing to us. It is stress in the widest sense, the inadequacy of our adjustability, that will become perhaps the most important disruptive influence in our society.

If I have today emphasized the applicability of animal behaviour research I do not want to be misunderstood. As in all sciences, applications come in the wake of research motivated by sheer intellectual curiosity. What this occasion enables me to emphasize is that biologically oriented research into animal behaviour, which has been done so far with very modest budgets, deserves encouragement, whatever the motivation and whatever the ultimate aims of the researcher. And we ethologists must be prepared to respond to the challenge if and when it comes.

REFERENCES

1. I call the method old because it must already have been highly developed by our ancestral hunter-gatherers, as it still is in non-westernized hunting-gathering tribes such as the Bushmen, the Eskimo, and the Australian Aborigines. As a scientific method applied to man it could be said to have been revived first by Charles Darwin in 1872 in *The Expression of the Emotions in Man and the Animals* (John Murray, London, 1872).

2. L. Levi, Ed., *Society, Stress, and Disease*, volume 1, *The Psychosocial Environment and Psychosomatic Diseases* (Oxford Univ. Press, London 1971).

3. The clearest introduction is: F. M. Alexander, *The Use of Self* (Chaterston, London, 1932); but a great deal of interest can also be found in: F. M. Alexander, *Man's Supreme Inheritance* (Chaterston, London, 1910) and *The Universal Constant in Living* (Chaterston, London, 1942).

4. The history of medical science is full of such examples of breakthroughs due to a reorientation of attention. Compare, for example, Jenner's discovery that milkmaids did not contract smallpox; Goldberger's observation that the staff of a "lunatic asylum" did not develop pellagra; Fleming's wondering about empty areas around the *Penicillium* in his cultures.

5. W. Barlow, *The Alexander Principle* (Gollancz, London, 1973).

6. J. Dewey, see, for example, introduction to F. M. Alexander, *The Use of Self* (Chaterston, London, 1932).

7. A. Huxley, *Ends and Means* (Chatto and Windus, London, 1937); "End-gaining and means-whereby," *Alexander, J.* 4, 19 (1965).

8. G. E. Coghill, "Appreciation: The educational methods of F. Matthias Alexander", in F. M. Alexander, *The Universal Constant in Living* (Dutton, New York, 1941).

9. R. A. Dart, *S. Afr. Med. J.* 21, 74 (1947); *An Anatomist's Tribute to F. M. Alexander* (Sheldrake Press, London, 1970).

10. C. S. Sherrington, *The Endeavour of Jean Fernel* (Cambridge Univ. Press, London, 1946); *Man on His Nature* (Cambridge Univ. Press, London, 1951).

11. E. von Holst and H. Mittelstaedt, *Naturwissenschaften* 37, 464 (1950).

12. N. Tinbergen, *Proc. Roy. Soc. Lond. Ser. B* 182, 385 (1973).

THIRTY-ONE

Instinct and Functioning in Health and Disease
by Dr Peter Macdonald

I HAVE WITHIN recent years been profoundly impressed by a new vista which seems to me to have been opened up by the work and writings of a layman—F. Matthais Alexander—with definite bearings upon the science and art of medicine. As Alexander's activities are almost unknown to the profession, although an appreciative review of his book, *Constructive Conscious Control of the Individual*, appeared in the *British Medical Journal* of 14 May 1924, and as I have come to the conclusion that there is a *prima-facie* case that his work is of first-class importance, and as, if this be so, investigation by the medical profession is imperative, I decided to make use of this occasion to attract the attention of some members of the profession to it, in the hope that some person or persons better qualified than I am to make such investigations may have their interest aroused.

Perhaps I can start best by telling you how Alexander began his own investigations. He is an Australian, and as a young man was a reciter, and had in Australia a great reputation as such, and as a Shakespearian actor. He lost his voice, having contracted what is sometimes called "clergyman's sore throat", presumably a chronic or sub-acute laryngitis. He did what any other man in like circumstances would have done—he consulted a laryngologist. The laryngologist did what any other laryngologist would have done—he sprayed his throat and gave him inhalations, and prescribed rest, etc.—and the throat recovered. Alexander accordingly gave another recital, but by the end of it his voice had again failed. He went back to the laryngologist, who was also a friend, who advised another course of the same treatment which had been successful before. Alexander said "No"; the laryngologist asked "Why?"—and I beg you to note the answer. That answer was: "Do you not see? I went into that room with my throat right, and I was able to recite. I came out of it with my throat wrong, and I was unable to recite. What caused the change from right to wrong? It must have been something I did. I will find out what it was that I had been doing wrong. When I have found out that I will cease to do it. When I have ceased to do it I will get my throat right, and I shall need neither your help nor that of anyone else."

Then followed months of patient research. Mainly in front of a looking-glass Alexander made observations of how he used his mechanism—not only how he conducted himself in using his voice, but how he conducted himself generally; how he used that mechanism to sit down on a chair, how he used that mechanism to get up out of a chair, how he used it to walk, how he used it to breathe, how he used it to stand up straight, to bend, to kneel; how, generally, he used himself in the ordinary activities of life.

You will note the use of the looking-glass. Why was this? It was because Alexander had then—although but vaguely—recognized that in man's evolution from the stable environment in which he had passed by far the longest period of his life to the recent rapidly changing environment of what we call civilization, his sensory appreciation (that is to say, the knowledge which he derives from his feelings of what he is doing) is unreliable; so that, for instance, when he thinks he is standing up straight—that is, lengthening his spine— he is often shortening it; when he thinks he is relaxing muscles he is often tensing them; when he thinks he is putting his head forward he is often putting it back—a vague recognition which his researches on himself, and subsequently on others, confirmed.

From these researches certain conclusions were arrived at, the following being the most important:

1 The first conclusion is that which I have indicated above— namely, that man's sensory appreciation is generally unreliable, particularly as regards knowledge acquired through the muscular sense. If Bain is right in his theory that of all our senses the muscular sense is the most important—that from it, for instance, we derive our ideas of space and time; that, for example, I do not see that the wall at the other end of the room is about twice as far away as the chair near the middle of the room, but that I acquire that knowledge largely by the different amount of muscular energy I have to expend in turning my eyes so that they converge on a spot on the wall from that expended when they converge on a spot on the chair, and from the different amount of similar energy I have to expend to focus each eye so that I can have a clear image of the wall in one case and of the chair in the other; and if it be further true that our sensory appreciation is unreliable, and that knowledge obtained through this sense is likewise unreliable, then civilized man is in a danger zone which will inevitably expose him to serious risks.

2 The second conclusion is that, generally speaking, in the ordinary activities of life man uses himself badly: that he does not know how to get up to the best advantage from a sitting to a standing position, nor how to stand up when he is standing, nor how to get down to a sitting from a standing position, nor how to continue to sit

I

down when he is down, nor how to walk to the best advantage, still less to run to the best advantage, or to inspire and expire to the best advantage. Now, though the importance of the proper performance of these several functions varies in degree, you will agree that some of these activities, or others cognate to them, are associated with everything man does—whether he is presiding at a meeting such as this, or leading a parliament, or writing a book, or teaching the young, or writing a play, or building a shop, or making a motor-car, or ploughing a field, or leading a strike. If Alexander is right, then, generally speaking, throughout his varied activities civilized man fails to function to the best advantage.

3 Man is a psycho-physical whole, and does not consist of mind and body, or of head and trunk and legs and lungs and heart and liver; he is a unified whole, and if a part seems to be defective the defect is probably one of the whole mechanism, and not of the part. Take, for instance, flat-foot. This is not a defect of the foot alone, the remedy for which is something dealing with the foot alone; it is the result of a defect in the use of the mechanism which controls the carriage of the whole body, and may be got rid of by the means which will rectify this faulty use.

4 Diseases are inseparable from wrong functioning, and in most of these wrong functioning is primary and disease secondary. Much disease can be prevented by the prevention of wrong functioning, and can be eliminated by the restoration of right functioning.

5 Man differs from the lower animals in that in their conduct instinct is the important guide, and reason plays a small part; in man's conduct instinct plays a smaller and reason a greater part. Instinct is the result of accumulated racial experiences. Man, in the process of leaving the tree and arriving in this twentieth century in London or York, has taken, say, a million years. For by far the largest part of that time he has been in a state of savagery, or pre-civilization, say, more than 990,000 years; for by far the smallest part he has been in a state of civilization. Instinct, accordingly, is more than 990,000 parts due to the experiences of the savage, less than 10,000 parts due to the experiences of civilization, and only infinitesimally due to the experiences of the civilization of the present day. Instinct, therefore, can be a sound guide to present conduct only if our experiences are similar to those of our ancestors. The experiences of our savage ancestors were acquired in a highly stable environment. Ours is a changing environment, and ever more rapidly changing; hence instinct has become, and is ever more and more becoming, an unsound guide to conduct, and it is ever becoming more and more

imperative that for it should be substituted a conscious control.

These are among the more important of Alexander's conclusions, and it is not my purpose today to attempt to prove them, or to claim that they are all of equal originality or importance. My object is solely to attract attention so that others may be interested to investigate; but I would like to refer specially to the second and fifth of these conclusions.

The second is that, generally speaking, man uses himself badly in the ordinary activities of life. I would ask you to make some observations on your friends who are over 50 years of age, or still more over 60, and I am prepared to wager that you will find that many of them have a waist measurement as large as, or larger than, their chest measurement, and you will find few in whom there is not present a stoop, with the chin thrown forward and head drawn back, with, if you try to move the head, an accompanying rigidity of the muscles of the head and neck, so that you will find difficulty in pushing the head on one side if you want to examine the ear. I do not believe that these manifestations are a result of old age; I believe that the misuse of the organism which brings them about constitutes one of the causes of it. Unfortunately, you find them in young people also, and, I think, increasingly so.

The second of the conclusions I wish to refer to is No. 5, and I will give two instances of how change of environment has converted a useful instinct into a harmful one, the second instance throwing some light, in my opinion, on why instinct, derived as it is from racial experience, tends to lessen health and promote disease.

(*a*) There is reason to believe that with primitive man, as is the case with many animals, the stranger was an enemy and was killed. This was generally an entirely reasonable process, and was arrived at from observations of experiences that if you did not kill him he killed you; or, where food supply was short, if he obtained the food you had to go without, and accordingly died. Though as regards persons this instinct has largely died out, and we now recognize that an advantage to one person does not necessarily or usually involve disadvantage to others, traces are left. *Hostis* is a Latin word with two meanings—the one is "stranger" and the other is "enemy"; and there used to be a tradition that there were villages where the normal thing to do to a stranger was to heave half a brick at him. But where the horde psychology comes into play this instinct still continues, and there are persons who still believe that one nation's advantage means the disadvantage of other nations, and we still have hostile action in various spheres between nation and nation or class and class.

(*b*) My second instance, however, is one with an important relation to the science and art of medicine. I have come to learn from Alexander that health is associated with a satisfactory use of the mechanism which controls the carriage of the body, and that this control should be such that the spinal column is maintained as erect as possible. In other words, the vertebrae should be pulled away from one another rather than pressed together through a co-ordinated use of the mechanism which tends to elongate rather than depress. More particularly the control of the neuromuscular mechanism should be such that the neck portion of the spinal column should be continued up as straight as possible, with the head square on top of it, throughout most of the activities of life. These words "straight" and "square" are used for the moment loosely, and I am aware that they need further definition, or, probably better, demonstration, as I shall indicate later in this paper.

Those of you who know the work of Professor Magnus of Utrecht, and who have read the most important lecture he delivered at Edinburgh on the physiology of posture, in which, for instance, he points out that in his experiments on "attitudinal reflexes" "the whole mechanism of the body acts in such a way that the head leads and the body follows", will see how the conclusion of Alexander as to the importance of the relation between head and neck, neck and trunk, is borne out by laboratory experiments. In fact, Alexander has in his work and in the technique he has devised for re-educating his pupils anticipated some of the results which Magnus and others have arrived at through these laboratory experiments.

If the use of the mechanism concerned with the control of the carriage of the body is thus satisfactory, the tension of the great abdominal muscles will not permit of the pendulous abdomen so often associated with age, with all its liability to visceroptosis and intestinal stasis.

Why is it the case that this right use and satisfactory carriage of the human body is rare? In my opinion it is due to the carrying over of a primitive instinct, which was once sound and helpful enough, into an environment where it has become unsound and harmful. The dominant factor of life in primitive man and the ancestors of primitive man must have been fear, and it is my belief that when man became *Homo sapiens* he dared not stand erect. If he raised himself erect he was liable to be seen over the shrubs or grass in which he stood by sabre-toothed tiger or wood wolf or cave bear, and accordingly eaten. Hence he learnt to crouch and peer with head thrown backwards and down. It was a habit for which there was then a sound reason. But this instinct has been carried over to civilization, where instead of being an advantage, it has become a disadvantage in the sedentary environment of modern life, with resulting flaccid muscles, pendulous belly, and accompanying conditions. This is surmise; but let me remind you of the reason given why a horse, when he gets up, rises on its fore feet and then on the hind, whereas the cow gets up first on the hind feet and then on the fore. The reason given is that in the environment of fear—which is the common ancestral environment of all animals, man included—the horse raised his head up before his body because he lived on grassy plains, and he raised his head above the grass to look over it for enemies before he showed himself fully; whereas the cow lived in the forest and kept its head low to the last so as to look for its enemies below the branches where it could see them best.

It is an accepted scientific opinion that at the present stage of the evolutionary process modern civilized man is in imperfect adjustment to his environment. The importance of Alexander's work lies in his emphasizing the reality of this maladjustment of man's neuro-muscular system, and in his having devised a technique for teaching pupils a right, or rather a better, use of themselves.

I cannot tell you much of the technique, for in the first place there is today no time, in the second I am not competent to do so, and in the third I am sceptical if it can be described in words. Words give such messages only from one brain to another as can be conveyed through the sense of hearing. Even the written word carries messages through the sense of hearing translated from the sense of sight. Words cannot be used to convey any meaning as to a sensory appreciation. You cannot really describe a colour in words so as to convey any meaning to another person unless he already knows the colour. Part of the technique, however, consists in the inhibition of wrong use. This is seldom easy, at least with adults. You all know how difficult it is to "keep the head down" at golf.

Another part is concerned with the method by which ends are attained. "Ends," says Alexander, "should not be arrived at direct." If the end is held in view successful attainment of the end is unlikely. Success is attained only by attention to the "means-whereby" that end can be reached. With correct attention to the "means-whereby" success in attaining the end is assured.

Let us again take a golf instance. I presume that there are few of you who have not had advice from a professional to "follow through" in driving a golf ball; and I am certain that no one of you ever met a professional who was able to tell you how to do it. In this, obviously, end-gaining gains no end; it only interferes with the attainment of the end desired.

If Alexander is right, then, the sound use of the mechanism and the elimination of instinct as a guide to that use is of first-class importance to all man's activities, and—what is of interest to us as a body of medical men—in the prevention of disease; and if it is as important as he says it is, his work should be incorporated in the education of our young, if only as a matter of preventive medicine.

Alexander is a teacher pure and simple. He does not profess to treat disease at all. If the manifestations of disease disappear in the process of education, well and good; if not, the education of itself will have been worth while. Manifestations of disease, however, do disappear. Including myself, I know many of his pupils—some of them, like myself, medical men. I investigated some of these cases, and I am talking about what I know. For instance, there was a case of flat-foot. Please note that Alexander was not directly interested in this foot. What he did was to teach the pupil how to use his brain and muscular mechanism in sitting down and getting up, how to comport his head in relation to his neck, his neck in relation to his thorax, his thorax in relation to his breathing, how generally to control the carriage of his body; and, in the process, not only the disabilities associated with dropped arches of the foot disappeared, but the dropped arches rose.

In other cases, under the like process, there seemed to be a distinct betterment in case of angina pectoris, of asthma, of epilepsy, of tremor, of spinal curavature, and of difficulty in walking from loco-motor ataxy, and from infantile paralysis. In short, I have seen, during the application of an educative process not directed to cure of disease, manifestations of disease disappear, so that I personally am convinced that Alexander is at least largely right when he says that disease is the result of wrong functioning. And further, I am begin-ning to wonder whether there are manifestations of any forms of chronic disease which may not disappear under a process of re-education on these lines, and whether McDonagh may not be right when he states in his great book that all disease is one; and whether the origin of that one disease does not lie in wrong functioning, and its different manifestations depend on different variations in functioning.

In conclusion, let me remind you again of my object in speaking to you. It is not, primarily, to communicate knowledge to you, but to endeavour to arrest the attention of some members of the medical profession to what I consider to be a most important development in connection with medicine. I am in hope that I have made out a *prima-facie* case for investigation by competent observers.

THIRTY-TWO

The Technique and Back Disorders
by Eric de Peyer

(A condensed version of the paper read by Mr de Peyer at a meeting of the Royal Society of Medicine on 22 November 1962)

THE SCOPE OF the Alexander Technique is so wide that it is easy to overlook its great potential value in solving specific therapeutic problems. The fact that it is primarily a re-educational procedure rather than directly medical, and is not concerned with fine differences of diagnosis, does not at all mean that even intractable symptoms may not disappear when the sufferer learns to apply Alexander's Principles.

If, as often happens, people have aches and pains which have defeated ordinary medical procedures, it may be because a habit of muscular tension and misuse has been formed which needs to be unlearned. A great deal of chronic backache is of this kind. The body will tolerate unfair pressures and faulty mechanics for a time, but often at middle age, or before, it begins to protest—sometimes violently. Heat treatment or manipulation may relieve the pain, but until the sufferer learns to use his back as nature intended, the relief is unlikely to be permanent. By means of the Alexander Technique good bodily usage can be restored, with the result that the relief of pain is more likely to be permanent.

Take, for instance, a typical case: a woman of 38 with chronic backache. The X-rays showed "arthritic changes" in the lumbar region. Physiotherapy was used, and quite effectively; the pain went. But temporarily only. More physiotherapy was used, with the same result. By chance she heard of the Alexander Technique and arranged to have some lessons. After only three it was quite apparent that the way she was holding herself had a great deal to do with the onset of pain. If the unnecessary tension was released and her back was no longer pulled in, the pain began to disappear. Soon she learnt to undo this tension for herself, and after the initial feeling of "unnaturalness", began to prefer using her back in this new way. As the habit of improved use became established, the pain steadily diminished, until it was wholly absent. No more physiotherapy was needed, and instead of "learning to live with her pain" and taking aspirins when it became too bad, she was able to live a free, normal, active life. This happened nearly ten years ago and she is still free of pain.

Exercises are often recommended as a way of changing faulty muscular habits. The reason why they are not effective takes us to the heart of Alexander's contribution to the story of human behaviour. We all have a way of using our bodies (in walking, sitting down, bending and so on) which is natural to us. Thus, we often recognize a friend at a distance by his stance or gait. It is very difficult to escape from this characteristic pattern of movement, because it would feel too odd and peculiar if we did. We subconsciously reject any way of using our bodies other than our own special way simply because we are used to it. The familiar feels "right" and the unfamiliar feels "wrong". Moreover our sense of security and balance is bound up with the maintenance of the customary feeling.

What happens if we do exercises? Naturally enough we do them in our own individual way. But if our doctor believes we need exercises it is highly probable that our own individual way is extremely faulty. Hence, what is to prevent us from performing our exercises in that same faulty style? If, for example, we normally stiffen our neck excessively in all activities, we shall certainly continue to do so while doing exercises. Or if we hollow our back habitually, we are not likely suddenly to stop doing so during our exercise period. A crooked man proverbially walks a crooked mile, but so also does a stiff-necked man or a hollow-backed man do a stiff-necked or hollow-backed exercise. We are to a large degree conditioned by our past habits and imprisoned in the muscular sets we have made for ourselves. What makes it so difficult to escape is that we are unaware of our state, and just as many people literally enjoy ill-health, so we, like the cage-bird, enjoy our captivity.

Alexander got round the problem of untrustworthy feeling by giving his pupils the experience of doing the ordinary, basic movements of everyday life without the habitual misdirection of energy and excessive tension or distortion of the bodily shape. He used his hands to do this, guiding them and undoing over-tension whenever it occurred, while their main concern was to be sure to switch off the urge to react in the same old automatic way. Unless the pupil made himself neutral and uncommitted, he could not receive the new muscular experience in a pure form; the old habit would still be operating to some extent. For in the attempt to change any habit, whether in the technique of piano-playing, or golf, or speech, or even merely sitting-down, no progress will be made unless the highest priority of all is given to the idea of change. As soon as this loses its priority, the pupil will inevitably revert to gaining his end in the old familiar way. This is what Alexander called "end-gaining". Crossing the road without looking is a simple example of "end-gaining" (and in modern conditions of traffic, end-gaining in possibly more than one sense!). But so is jumping to a wished-for conclusion without passing through any logical train of evidence. Stammerers are obvious end-gainers, because they try very hard to speak using the wrong means of clenched jaw and tense lips. (I am not, of course, suggesting this is all there is to stammering.)

The principles on which the Alexander Technique is based do not in any way conflict with accepted anatomical and physiological knowledge. It is known that the human body functions best if the spine is normally kept extended and that habitual over-tension not only constricts the blood vessels and reduces respiratory efficiency but tends to distort the body as well.

There is another point that is sometimes forgotten. Good muscular habits maintain the natural margin of safety. For example, the spinal vertebrae become better spaced, so that impingement on nerve trunks by displacement becomes less likely. Stepping unexpectedly off a pavement is far more liable to have serious consequences if one's spine is habitually badly aligned than if good postural habits normally keep the vertebrae in their proper position.

Bad use therefore increases accident-proneness. We become more vulnerable because our bony structure has no margin of error. We cannot afford to make a false move.

The same principle applies in a more psychological sense. If we are habitually strung up, the inevitable irritations, frustrations, disappointments (not to mention the real disasters) of life become intolerable burdens. We have no safety margin to take any extra load. Hence, one can perhaps say that far more important than the kind of misfortunes in a person's life is the sort of state he is in when they occur. If we are tense, small things seem unbearable, and molehills become mountains. If we are not tense, there is at least more chance that we can bear them philosophically and adapt ourselves. I am not suggesting that there is no more to the problem than comparative degrees of tension. It isn't nearly so simple as that, because we are all largely conditioned by our past experience working on our character and temperament. But I do say that the same person, given his (perhaps) peculiar psychology, will react very differently to the same sort of stimulus at different times.

Certain bodily habits go with certain mental habits. Depression is a literal physical fact, as well as a mental one. Hence, if we habitually adopt a depressed posture, we are already depression-prone.

Take one more case, a man in the middle 40s. He had been through the whole gamut of medical treatment, and reckoned altogether he had spent £1,000 in trying to get cured. He had his teeth out, had spinal manipulation from orthopaedists, manipulation also from three different osteopaths, was examined with negative results for diabetes, kidney trouble and a TB spine, and was advised to wear a steel corset. All this was backed by scores of X-ray photographs. He had not omitted to consult a psychologist and had even tried the Black Box.

When he came to me he was quite desperate, indeed almost suicidal. For it was no ordinary backache, but one that extended down his legs to his feet and produced a most unpleasant muzzy feeling in his head.

At the first lesson, we made good progress and he went away much encouraged. At the second, he said excitedly, "I think we've got it!" I, too, was excited, because it was becoming obvious that he only needed to be released from tension for all his pain to disappear. Owing to a bad fall he had had, his muscles had gone into a protective spasm, as if to prevent his being hurt again, and this had become fixated, so that he had lost all power of recapturing normal feeling. What he needed, and what no other treatment had given him, was to be *given* the experience of normal feeling instead of the tense, perverted muscular sensations he had got used to.

After that second lesson he went home, went to bed at 6 pm and slept without waking till 8 o'clock the next morning. From then on the problem was more or less solved. With more lessons he got increased confidence in his ability to put himself right, and he describes the change that occurred (now eight years ago) as a "fantastic transformation".

Can all back troubles be cured by the Alexander Technique? Of course not. For there are a few back disorders in which muscular tension and bad body mechanics are not a significant factor, and which require medical treatment. On the other hand, it would be a pity to undergo dangerous and useless operations, or to let pain and discomfort spoil years of one's life, or even to spend £1,000 on medical tests and treatments, before finding out that the real way to better health lies through re-education.

THIRTY-THREE

Medical Aspects of the Alexander Technique
by Dr Wilfred Barlow
(A lecture given at the Alexander Institute in 1965)

IT IS ASTONISHING to me that I should not have found it easy to produce for you tonight a large number of doctors who could talk to you knowledgeably about the Alexander Technique. This would not have been the case in the days prior to world war II. When I first got to know Alexander in 1937, he was very much inclined to orientate his work towards medicine. He had come to this country from Australia, armed with letters of introduction from several doctors, and although he soon made most of his impact on the theatrical profession, a selection of "letters-of-approval" which had been written by various famous actors and actresses and which he printed as an advertisement, showed that almost all of these notable people were expressing gratitude for his help with their medical problems —usually breathing disorders, colds, catarrh, vocal difficulties and so on. He himself was delighted when several doctors wrote to the *British Medical Journal* on 29 May 1937 applauding his work, and he would write to—and occasionally get published in—other medical journals such as the *Lancet*. At his 80th dinner party in 1949, the top table consisted in the main of members of the medical profession, plus Sir Stafford and Isobel Cripps, and a professor of Scientific Method, Professor Heath. It was only after the shock of the South African libel action that those around him appeared to have become frightened at the vulnerability of some of his more extravagant medical claims, and in the 1950s, it began to be put about that his technique did not belong in medicine, but was to be seen as basically concerned with education. In fact, since Alexander died in 1955, the medical implications of the Alexander Principle have been ridiculously underplayed by the majority of Alexander teachers, except for those who work at the Alexander Institute. So, before I embark on pointing out why the medical implications of the Alexander Principle are so important, let me have a crack at the "educationalists".

F. M. Alexander came to this country in 1904. About 30 years later, in 1932, a course for the training of teachers in his method was started. Yet here we are, in 1965, over 30 years later—60 years in fact since Alexander came to this country—and what have we got to show for it educationally? Precisely one small infant school of, it is hoped, eight children—please do not think I am decrying this valuable venture—but let us see that this is a very small egg indeed to roll out of a 60-year-old elephant.* The story repeats itself again and again— high educational ideals only rarely finding practical expression—and whilst we must admire the efforts of some of the earlier teachers, what are we to say of an educational approach in which "non-doing" so easily becomes "nothing-doing", and in which inhibition becomes unresponsiveness.

There seems to me to be a deep-seated malaise in the present Alexander preoccupation with education, and I want to try to get to the bottom of this quite false split between the educational and medical approach.

Please don't get me wrong. Of course I see that the technique is, in its moment-to-moment practice and application, an educational technique and not a curative technique: but I wonder how many people here can lay their hands on their hearts, and say that they have not been interested by its health aspect, by its influence on their own health, mental and physical. What Alexander and many of his teachers were frightened of, I think, was this. So many techniques and methods exist in which something is done *to* the patient, without any attempt being made to teach the patient. The word "patient" indeed conjures up the idea of someone who is a passive recipient of whatever the doctor may think fit to do. It conjures up the idea of, say, manipulation, massage, laying on of hands, hypnosis, behaviour therapy, grateful mums with tears in their eyes, of treating people as the poor dears who aren't very intelligent, the Poor Law sick, rows of mental beds wired up for shock therapy, tranquillized businessmen groping for pep pills to break out temporarily from their drugged state of calm, and so on and so on. Or to put it briefly, the Alexander teacher rightly refuses to see his pupil as a mechanism, he wishes to see him as a person.

Now comes the next step in the Alexandrian's thought. What he sees in a flash is this: that if analysis into mechanism leads to treating people as de-humanized conglomerations of molecules and cells and tissues, then this is not for him. And what is more, any *explanation* in

* Since I wrote this this small school has disappeared but in recent years the ILEA have started to give grants for people to train to become Alexander teachers: it should be pointed out that these grants were first given to the Alexander Institute on the basis of the *medical* and scientific research which had been carried out there.

terms of mechanism is not for him either: and the argument goes on that since the doctors and the physiologists and so on work on the basis of analysing their patients into bits and pieces, nothing they can offer can add to the Alexander teacher's skill.

It seems to me vital to clear up this muddle. It is basic to the relationship of the Alexander Technique to medicine and, whilst the muddle persists, I cannot see how the new teachers we are training now can avoid getting stuck in the same old Alexander rut. So I want to talk about *explanation* and, in particular, just where scientific explanation fits in with our work, and why medical knowledge is a help. Firstly, let me put forward some of the arguments which I have heard Alexander teachers make against explanation.

Firstly, it is said that Alexander himself thought it unnecessary to have theoretical knowledge of this kind—he castigated in his books an anatomist who, with all his anatomical knowledge, nevertheless manifested an appalling misuse in his own body.

Secondly, the general philosophy of Holism says that "we murder when we dissect". It says that if we pull up a plant by its roots to see how it grows, it dies: that when we analyse the human body we will only find what we look for: that the ways in which we look at the human body—and the instruments we use to do this looking—determine what we will find. This argument was well put by the biologist Claude Bernard—here is a well-known passage from his *Milieu Interne*. "In the living thing, there are two orders of phenomenon, firstly, the phenomenon of vital creation or of organic synthesis: secondly the phenomenon of death or vital destruction." He went on to castigate those who seek to promote life by studying the second procedure: "When they wish to designate phenomena of life, they are really speaking of phenomena of death." In much the same way Alexander philosophy has said that a fragmentary approach to the human organism contributes nothing to the vital teaching process.

Thirdly, it is quite clear that in the first half of the twentieth century modern medicine went crazy in its preoccupation with detail. The discovery of the microscope and of new techniques of biochemistry and biophysics led to the body being cut up and analysed into smaller and smaller pieces, so that the doctor gets to know more and more about less and less, and so that each organ comes to have its own type of doctor, who, because of the immensity of the detail he has to learn, knows little even of what his other medical colleagues know, and loses sight of the care of the whole person— "the operation was successful, but the patient died" and so on.

Fourthly, it is said that time spent on explaining is a waste of previous Alexander teaching time which should be spent during the Alexander lesson in giving the "Alexander experience": and as part of this argument, it is said that once a pupil starts talking and discussing things, he will employ just those bad habits which we are trying to stop. Some Alexander teachers are reputed to reply, "You stiffened your neck when you asked that question."

Finally I am sure you can all of you think of many more reasons why medical and physiological knowledge should not be injected into Alexander's work—that there is a vast amount of it and that to acquire it properly would need a disproportionate amount of time: that anatomists and physiologists make it their business to *describe* the various conditions of structure and function, but that our concern, as teachers, is to *bring about* healthy functioning rather than to describe it.

I am only too well aware of these basic arguments and I am sympathetic with those who hold them strongly, but most of those who decry explanation, be it anatomical, physiological, psychological, behavioural or philosophical—are in fact themselves already using many forms of explanation. Alexander himself used whatever bits of anatomy and physiology he could get hold of—Magnus's Zentralapparat, Sherrington's concept of the integrative action of the nervous system and of the inhibitory state, Coghill's total pattern concept, plus anatomical terms used with puzzling inaccuracy—the knee, for example, is an ill-defined anatomical point, the "back" is vague and puzzling to many people, Alexander's head-neck relationship at one point may seem to involve the skull on the first cervical vertebra, at another time the skull and neck on the dorsal spine. Constantly, I am meeting with Alexander pupils who are not only confused about the directions they are being given but have little notion about the actual forms of misuse which they themselves manifest. Far from it being the case that Alexander himself did not delve into detail, he only came across his discoveries by the most minute examination of detail. As Bernard Shaw put it: "Alexander is calling on the world to witness a change which he alone can see"—and when we come to consider the relationship between the manner of use and the various forms of disease, it is only by a most accurate analysis of each pupil's particular manifestations that we can give all the help that is needed and begin to see why it is that one pupil manifests one particular form of malfunctioning whilst another pupil manifests another. It is inescapable that Alexander himself had a theoretical framework, and that he used anatomy—sometimes rather inaccurate anatomy.

It frequently happens that teachers are not able to alter a pupil's manner of use because the actual physical conditions don't respond according to the simplified anatomical scheme which Alexander put forward. Alexander and some of his teachers have blamed this failure on what amounts to a moral lack—debauched kinaesthesia, endgaining, refusal to inhibit, and so on: but some years ago I met a pupil who had had a stormy session of teaching with an Alexander teacher who had reduced her to tears because she would not react as he wished. When she saw her doctor soon afterwards she was found to have a fractured pelvis. She was elderly with very brittle bones. This is a gross example and it is not in any way suggested that her pelvis was fractured during the lesson, but it indicates that it is essential to know something of the physical and psychological factors which limit a pupil's trainability at any given time. And again, I have for some time pointed out a ridiculous error which appeared in a paper by an Alexander teacher which shows X-rays of a neck "before" and "after" making an Alexander adjustment. In the "improved" X-ray, the neck has been so over-straightened that one of the vertebrae in the middle of the neck has been displaced slightly forward on the one below it. There is already a tendency to mock at the improved Alexander use of the neck and head as being over-stiff and over straight such an X-ray does not help this impression.

The second point which I raised as being a contraindication to detailed anatomical and physiological knowledge is the Holistic argument. This is the belief that analysis of structure is unnecessary, that when we drive a car, what we need to know is how to control it rather than how the actual mechanical engineering of the car works. Yet we must remember that as teachers we are dealing with human cars, which have blocked carburettors, noisy exhausts and very bad brakes. When a car goes wrong it is necessary to have an engineer in addition to someone to teach us to drive. Certainly, we can learn to drive without knowing anything about the engine. This is fine until the engine goes wrong. This argument between Holism and mechanism is the same argument as that between analysis and synthesis which pervades much philosophical thought at present. André Gide seemed to have the meat of the matter when he said that "Analysis must always precede synthesis, but all the preparatory work must be re-absorbed: it must become invisible although always there."

The third objection which I raised was that medicine has gone crazy in its preoccupation with cells and tissues, with the pathological organ rather than with the person. Nevertheless, it is necessary for Alexander teachers to know to what extent changes in the body are reversible and to what extent irreversible. An amputated leg cannot be put back. Many diseases are almost as irreversible as an amputation, and like the amputation, all we can promise is to teach people to improve the rest of themselves and not to deteriorate generally because of the stimulus of their disorder. It is cruel to raise false hopes, but it is also good medicine to indicate just how much can be done to add "life to the years".

As I pointed out in my fourth objection, it is said that time spent on explaining is wasted. This in my experience is never the case. Sooner or later with each pupil we run into resistance. Each pupil requires talking to in a language he can accept. If we are clever, we can forestall the questions the pupil will inevitably ask by answering them beforehand in the early honeymoon stage of lessons where the pupil listens avidly to almost everything we say. As one gets more skilled in teaching, one learns to know the sorts of arguments which certain people will eventually throw up, and by providing explanations before people want them, we can avoid emotional set-to's: and by having ourselves thought out clearly the sorts of problems that the technique touches on, we can teach much more confidently.

The last argument was that it takes too much time to learn enough to be able to give such adequate explanation. I think the answer lies with all of us, that we need a good explanatory framework for our Alexander Technique. Alexander's creative-evolution theories are fine for many people but may scare others off. In order to understand fully what people in the past have said, we always have to interpret them in terms of our modern knowledge, just as we ourselves know that every single day, if we are to be and to know what we are, we have to find out repeatedly again and again what we are. The sort of new theoretical framework which will constantly have to be built, year in and year out, for the Alexander Technique, is required for two interlocking reasons: so that we can explain things to our pupils in the language of their times, and so that we can understand ourselves what we are teaching and what we have been taught. Informed discussion as a preliminary will gain the pupil's co-operation. When he then directs his head "forward-and-up" it will be for the right reason. It is my firm belief that we may get people free and using themselves well, but if they get this improved manner of use for the *wrong* reasons it will eventually go bad on them.

Often indeed we hear that an Alexander lesson may be given without any explanation at all, and that all that matters is the "experience". Yet surely the danger here is that the teaching is becoming a form of passive therapy rather than an education. Surely it is the explaining and teaching part of the lesson which prevents it deteriorating into mere manipulation, however skilled that might be. Or again, if the application of the Alexander Technique is measured by the ability of one person to work with or on another person, then this too loses the whole point, which is to equip a pupil to work on himself, when he is away from the lesson. In my practice, I define a patient as someone who cannot yet be expected to help himself: a pupil as someone who is ready to take responsibility for his own misuse. There is in the most desperate cases usually a small area where responsibility can be taken immediately, but many of us remain a mixture of *patient* and *pupil* for a long time, before proceeding to the desired next stage of being an individual *person* who needs neither treating nor teaching.

What I am trying to get the discussion round to is the point of view that just because we may use the technique in dealing with medical patients, this does not mean that it is not an educational technique. On the contrary, the sick human being requires a great deal of explanation and needs teaching *what* as well as teaching *how*. It is precisely the quality of our theoretical explanatory framework which will make our technique an educational rather than a curative technique. So far from ill people considering it as a form of therapy, most of them see only too clearly that they must re-educate themselves, and the stimulus of ill-health makes most of them work much harder than, say, the adolescent schoolboy who has been detailed off to have lessons by his parents or his school. Only the teacher is to blame if what he does with people is regarded by them as a cure.

What Sorts of Medical Conditions?

I want to switch from this to a consideration of the sorts of medical conditions which can be dealt with by the Alexander Technique of re-education. I am repeatedly asked, as I am sure many of you are, "What conditions can be helped?" The quick answer "almost all conditions", although true, is not very helpful—what we are concerned with is which particular conditions are really crying out for knowledge and application of Alexander's principles. The conditions which I mention are those which I myself have seen helped in this way, and those in which there seems to be a connection between misuse and malfunctioning. To establish statistically the extent to which Alexander's principles are needed in such conditions is a matter for research workers in the future—I can myself only state what, in my work as a clinician, I have found to be the case, and such an opinion is, of course, only as good as my own clinical standing as a consultant in the NHS. In the past, funds have not been made available for research although only a modest outlay now would, I am convinced, produce large dividends.

1 Gynaecological Conditions

The technique has been found by many people to be useful in child-birth, both in the pre-natal, natal, and post-natal phases. There are many techniques at present which teach relaxation and breathing techniques and in my experience the Alexander Technique is usually sufficient without the need for other forms of training.

I have mentioned in my book, *The Alexander Principle*, that many women, around the time of the menopause, find that the stabilization of their "body-image" (which comes from doing Alexander work) is something to hold on to at a time when their general bodily feelings are becoming different and often muddled. I should perhaps also mention "period-pains" which are often alleviated by the general release of tension and alteration in pelvic attitude which follows re-education. And this list would not be complete if I did not mention that the sensitivity of the Alexander teacher's hands in adjusting the pupil's body have often led to the detection of tumours, whether they be uterine or ovarian, which have previously passed unnoticed. The Alexander teacher would, of course, only comment on the discovery of something which felt unusual and immediately recommend consulting the patient's doctor.

2 Disorders of the Digestive Tract

The digestive tract is particularly prone to the various stress diseases which affect our modern civilization, whether it be gastric and duodenal ulcers, spastic colon, or ulcerative colitis. Again, the mechanism for relief of symptoms is simply one of teaching the patient to adapt to stress: and one should point out that many pains are referred to the abdomen by nerve pressure from the vertebral column or else from muscular spasm in the back or in the abdominal wall.

3 Disorders of the Heart and Blood Vessels

As a general principle, it is clear that the more economically the body is used, the less strain will be put on the heart. As with abdominal pains, many chest pains are caused by nerve pressure from the dorsal spine and it is astonishing how many doctors and consultants fail to notice quite marked deformities in the dorsal spine and chest cage.

It is interesting that the incidence of coronary thrombosis is much higher on a Monday morning after a weekend and clearly there must be some disorder of adaptation in this fact. I have never found a patient yet who, having had a coronary, does not have an extremely fixed upper chest in front, and I regard it as of paramount importance that such patients should be taught to release this chest tension and learn to breathe properly according to Alexander principles. Conditions of high blood pressure also can often be alleviated by learning to use the body in a less tense manner and one should also mention the common symptoms of "poor circulation"—cold fingers and so on, which so many people complain of and which often clear up after re-education.

4 Sexual Disorders
I have discussed at length in *The Alexander Principle*, in a chapter entitled "The Psycho-Mechanics of Sex", the important part which muscular tension plays in sexual disorder: and likewise the important part which muscular homeostasis plays in giving a satisfactory sexual experience.

5 Breathing Disorders
I have found the technique extremely helpful in treating asthma and chronic bronchitis—in fact in any chest condition in which the patient needs to be taught to breathe more adequately.

6 Neurological Disorders
In the main the Alexander Technique is useful in the *rehabilitation* phase of the chronic neurological disorders, but more specifically I have found it helpful in treating trigeminal neuralgia, epilepsy, migraine, and torticollis. Obviously the neurological conditions which may come from obstruction to nervous pathways—such as cervical myelopathy or the giddiness which comes from vertebral artery spasm—will be helped by a re-education of vertebral balance.

7 Rheumatic Disorders
It is perhaps in this field that the Alexander Technique is most obviously and immediately useful, whether it be in the treatment of disc lesions of the neck and back, or for the more common low-back pain, which appears to have no obvious pathology. Osteo-arthritic conditions of the neck, back, hip and knee can often be helped as can such irritating disorders as tennis elbow and "frozen shoulder".

Obviously postural disorders will be greatly helped, and rheumatoid arthritis may be benefited by teaching the patient how to adapt to stress and to release tension.

8 Mental Health

I have found the Alexander Technique more useful in the psycho-neuroses—states of anxiety and depression, phobias, hysterical tics and odd movement patterns—than in psychotic states.

I am aware that this brief list of medical conditions is extremely superficial but it may at least suggest to doctors who are unable to help some of their patients in these categories, that it might be worth, in Professor Tinbergen's words, giving Alexander a try. The rationale for the medical use of the Alexander Technique has been given in my book, *The Alexander Principle*, and the field is now wide open for enterprising research students to establish the exact place which the technique should take up in the medical curriculum.

OBJECTIONS

Introduction

THE SELECTION OF essays in this book may give the impression that there has always been complete unanimity of opinion about the value of the Alexander Technique. There was always plenty of criticism of his work during his lifetime and there still is. In his lifetime the usual criticism was that his writings were obscure, difficult and repetitive—impossible to understand without personal lessons. And even with personal lessons, many still found the teaching difficult. This general bafflement was expressed in an article in the *Morning Post* of 7 March 1907, soon after the 38-year-old Alexander had come to England from Australia:

It may be (1) a defect in the intelligence of the reader, or (2) a defect in the literary power of the writer, or (3) a defect in the method itself (that is there may be no method at all), or it may be (4) a moral defect in Mr Alexander and he may not wish to be explicit: but it leaves the critic wondering whether the victim of his criticism is (1) a quack with a true method which he keeps secret, (2) a quack with a false method which cannot be explained, (3) a genius with a true method which he has not the literary power to make clear, or (4) a genius with a true method which none but a like genius could understand from the printed page. These four are all possible alternatives which it would be polite to mention and those who think they will be better able to choose among them than the present critic are welcome to their fancy.

Even such well-wishers as Archbishop Ramsay managed to give with one hand and take away with the other.

The great discovery of F. M. Alexander as to the direction of the whole human organism, though hailed as valuable by some of the most brilliant minds of our time—such men as Sir Charles Sherrington, Archbishop William Temple, Bernard Shaw, Lord Lytton, Aldous Huxley—has failed, so far, to find adequate philosophical and theological interpretation. The form of Alexander's writing is as dreadful as its content is valuable. Never has a true sage presented himself so well disguised as a commonplace, pretentious bore obsessed by fixed ideas.

These critical attacks on Alexander came to a head in an article published by the South African government in the 1940s, written in such offensive terms that Alexander had no alternative but to sue them. The summary of the Judgment which was published in the *Lancet* after Alexander had won his case gives an indication of the malevolent tone of some of this early criticism—the summary is published as chapter 35 since it was an important hurdle which Alexander's work had to overcome.

The early Alexander teachers survived this and much more of it, confident in the validity of their own practical approach, and they have arrived now, in the last quarter of the twentieth century, with a large and increasing demand for their services. No account of Alexander would be complete though if it did not mention the almost constant argumentation which has gone on and still goes on between Alexander teachers—some of it, no doubt, due to rivalry, some of it due to the economic facts of life: but whatever the reasons, the continual argumentation is indicative of considerable differences between teachers—my article on "Medical Aspects" (chapter 33) is a case in point. Whilst only too aware of my own medical bias, I have suggested in chapter 36 just why Alexander teaching may vary so much from one particular practitioner to another. Objections and criticisms are, however, the lifeblood of our work, just as they are in any other developing scientific discipline, and Dr Robin Skynner's article (chapter 34) on "The First Twelve Lessons" is a good example of the constructive criticism which we need.

THIRTY-FOUR

The First Twelve Lessons
by Dr Robin Skynner

THESE NOTES ARE simply an attempt to set down, after a dozen lessons in the Alexander Technique, the impressions I have formed so far of the aims of this training, and my present evaluations of the methods employed. No doubt I shall want to revise or withdraw many of these comments and criticisms when I have got a little further with the training and come to see the purpose of details, which are not significant to me now. But it will be useful to me to try to formulate my present ideas about it, if only so that I may be able to put my questions in a sufficiently clear form for you to be able to give me the answers I want. And what I have to say may be of interest as an example, at least, of the misconceptions newcomers are likely to acquire when they encounter the technique, and might suggest to you some precautionary measures that might be taken to avoid them.

1 The Presentation of the Aims of the Method
The impression I had of the aims of the method, and of the claims made for it, at least until after I had James Harvey Robinson's and Dewey's papers, was roughly this: That in man many of the activities that in animals are carried out by instinctive inborn patterns, have to be learned. This brings with it a great increase in the modifiability of behaviour, and so greater potentialities for new development, but carries with it the requirement that these activities require investigation to find the optimum method of performance, and then need to be learned just as one needs to learn to use a typewriter. We have not formerly realized this, and have assumed that we know how to do these things automatically. Because of this, we simply pick up the habits we see in our parents, or develop haphazard ourselves, habits which in fact are not those demanded by optimum efficiency and are often pernicious in their consequences. These habitual reactions are below the threshold of consciousness (i.e. we are not aware of the muscular movements involved in sitting down; we only know that we decide to do so and that we eventually arrive in the chair). They feel comfortable because we are used to them, and their ill-effects only become apparent to us via their consequences—feeling of ill-health, backaches and so on.

So far I could not agree more, and my interest in Alexander was aroused at first because he appears to have some method of attacking this. The method seemed to have as its basis the establishment of a certain dynamic relationship between the head and neck; this once established, other postural dynamics tended to right themselves. This did not seem unreasonable. The organism is intricately interrelated, and change in one part might be expected to bring about changes throughout the whole system if the alteration were made at some key position.

So far the whole thing seemed perfectly plausible. I found it much more difficult to stomach the claims that were made for the benefits accruing from this re-training. I could well imagine that the improved neuro-muscular functioning that might come about through the re-education could lead to an improvement in one's general feeling of health, one's cheerfulness, vigour and so on. One feels better when one takes exercise. But the claims seemed to go much further than that. I cannot remember very exactly the statements I've read in the papers and booklets you've given me, but the general burden of them appeared to be that Alexander had provided a means whereby human psychological reactions could be radically transformed. (You might object, quite justifiably, to the word psychological here; I am using it only to emphasize the "psycho" aspect of "psycho-physical", and to refer to such human behaviour, or such aspects of human behaviour, as we normally include under such classifications as "judgement", "thought", "emotional attitudes" and so on.) It was put forward as a competitor to psychoanalysis.

In other circumstances (if, for instance, I had read an article about Alexander by some author unknown to me) these claims would probably have inclined me against investigating further had my interest already been aroused almost to the point of doing so. It all seems too good to be true, or rather too improbable to believe. This is, of course, no criticism of the fact that these claims are made; I simply mention it because sometimes a new work can seem to be too good to be accepted and my experience is that it pays to make minimum claims or to present at first only some of the benefits it should make possible. Most of the writings have a "Christian Science" atmosphere about them, and I think this must deter many people from accepting the stuff.

I was, however, prepared to accept all this tentatively, and I was anxious to discover by what means these desirable ends might be brought about. The theory seemed to be that the neck-head relationship brought it about by some mysterious means which were labelled "the primary control". I say mysterious because in nothing I read did there appear to be any description or theory of how these various changes were related, of how a change in the head-neck relation could so profoundly affect man's "psychological" activities. And I use the word "labelled" deliberately because the term appeared to add nothing to the bare statements that the head-neck relation exercised a profound influence.

The only other hint I could find in the things I read as to the rationale of the method was in the discussions about "end-gaining" and "means-whereby". This meant very little to me. I found Alexander's explanations extremely difficult to follow, and found it as difficult to see any connection between this (means-whereby versus end-gaining) and the claimed "psychological" benefits as I did with the "primary control". Since there were no theoretical arguments for assuming that the training would lead to the benefits expected, decision on these claims had to be on wholly empirical grounds.

Now this is no way diminishes the correctness of Alexander's claims. If his methods will do what he says they will do, that's that. But it does diminish the chances of other people taking the claims seriously and investigating them. There are any number of cults and quacks promising the earth as a result of some kind of hocus pocus, and one hasn't the time to go around and check up on them all. One has to decide, therefore, on theoretical grounds which ones appear most plausible on the basis of the knowledge we have, and investigate them. An adequate theoretical basis for his methods would therefore make it more readily acceptable. Perhaps more important still, it should suggest new possibilities of experiment in the methods and perhaps enable them to be improved or augmented.

2 The Theory

I have already outlined my impressions of Alexander's theories, or rather my inability to discover any adequate ones. (I must admit I haven't looked very far, but I'm merely trying here to set down my present ideas.) What follows is therefore an attempt to fit such as I have acquired about the method and its consequences into my present knowledge; to formulate a theory that would explain to my own satisfaction the achievements of the method without conflicting with or going outside my current conceptions.

Now it seems to me that Alexander's methods are aimed at accomplishing two aims, which are more conveniently discussed separately:

1 More effective "postural dynamics" to attain optimally efficient action, with resulting improvement in health, feelings of well-being, lessened fatigue, etc.

2 Greater control of *all* reactions to stimuli (i.e. those reactions I have labelled "psychological" above as well as those one might call "postural") through an enhanced ability to inhibit automatic, habitual, unconscious patterns of behaviour and a consequent opportunity to substitute new, conscious, deliberate patterns.

These two aims are intimately connected but I think it is useful to distinguish them. In the training you appear to aim principally at replacing faulty postural dynamics by patterns more appropriate to our needs. This, however, cannot be done directly, because the faulty patterns of movement are initiated by deeply-ingrained, habitual chains of neural impulses normally below the threshold of consciousness. The chain is triggered off by a conscious awareness of a desired "end", but the rest of the chain, which is the content I ascribe to the term "means-whereby" at the moment, then goes forward as automatically as a patella-jerk after the blow with the hammer. We don't sit down unless we decide to, and so trigger off the chain, but once we have done so the chain continues and is beyond our control. It is thus necessary to inhibit this automatic response, and to start all over again building up a new chain, or "means-whereby", this time keeping the process conscious. Inhibition of the unconscious, and so uncontrollable, chains which determine our accustomed "postural dynamics" is thus a prerequisite if new, conscious chains are to be laid down, so that "2" above, in a limited sense, is the first requirement if "1" is to be achieved.

Now though Alexander is mainly concerned with training people to inhibit those automatic responses that I would describe as "postural", there seems no reason to me why the effects should be confined to just these responses. It may well be that the technique you are using (of giving stimuli like "sit down" and giving the pupil practice in not responding) is in effect developing just that general capacity to inhibit automatic responses and so achieving a "delayed reaction". This would provide a satisfactory explanation (at least for me) of the "psychological" improvements that are said to follow Alexander's training and which I find difficult to connect with the head-neck relation or with any improvement in "postural dynamics" alone. I fully agree that intellectual instruction alone will not alter emotional responses: clear thinking generally is by itself of little value, for one may think sanely enough while one is *trying* to apply new techniques; but as soon as one forgets to apply them, or meets a situation to which one's "emotional" responses are strong, one's habitual patterns of responses are triggered off before there is time for the new knowledge to be applied to the situation. Most of the foolish things men do are not just due to incorrect or inadequate information, which could be put right by a course of lectures or by reading a book, but are rather determined by deeply-ingrained, habitual patterns of evaluation passed on, without being consciously formulated, from generation to generation. The patterns of evaluation, or habits of thinking-and-feeling, or ways of reacting to stimuli in general, are largely unconscious, and so inaccessible to conscious alteration. We don't know we have them, just as the man-in-the-street is unaware that he is using Aristotelian logic, and so it never occurs to us to question them.

So much for (2). About (1) I have a good deal less to say that might be of interest to you. But I might as well summarize my interpretation of what you are trying to do in establishing the new head-neck-back relationship, so that you may see why I make the comments below on the practical technique. That a certain invariant relation in the head-neck-back complex should favour optimally efficient "body mechanics" I am simply prepared to accept. I know far too little about this to make any useful comment on why it should be so. But the suggestion you have made, e.g. that since the main sense organs, including the semicircular canals, are in the head, the head-neck adjustments should occupy first place in the neural "commands" which initiate bodily movements, seem perfectly reasonable.

As to the methods you use to train pupils in this new manner of use, I gather that you are trying (apart from developing the ability to inhibit the old patterns) to:

(a) Manipulate the body into the desired positions while the subject repeats a sequence of orders, and so set up a simple conditioned reflex. If a person can, by shining a light into his eye while repeating the word "contract", establish a reflex whereby the pupil automatically contracts when the word is uttered or thought of, one should certainly be able to set up a reflex of this kind. The number of repetitions employed in your training is, I think, of the order required to do this. I imagine that this is the reason why Alexander insists that as long as one gives the orders one cannot go wrong, since one's new reflex knows where one's head ought to be even better than one's re-educated kinaethesia.

(b) Re-educate the kinaesthetic sense. It would be impossible to *tell* someone how to get the desired head-neck-back relation. Since he has never experienced it, he has no symbols associated with it that you could use. While training him in a reflex reaction to the commands, you necessarily also get him to associate the descriptions "head forward and up" and so on with the appropriate set of sensations. This is perhaps not so important as training in the reflex, as far as the head-neck-back relation is concerned, but at the same time as you are laying this down you appear to be trying to educate the student into an awareness of the degree of muscular tension throughout his body, and by repeated adjustments, pointed out each time, to teach him to use the optimum tension throughout.

Assuming that these are the aims, the pupil should, presumably, first inhibit his response to the stimulus given by the instructor. This gives him practice in inhibiting the old habits. He should then allow the instructor to manipulate his body into the desired positions, repeating the appropriate verbal instructions, but without making any movements himself, and then maintain that adjustment until the instructor changes it. And finally, he should focus his attention on the adjustments the instructor makes to his legs, arms etc., while maintaining his awareness of the head-neck-back sensations.

3 The Practical Work

I think it would have assisted me if I had had some explanation on the lines of the above. Towards the end of the second week I found myself getting quite frustrated because I found it so difficult to understand what was required of me. Reading in James Harvey Robinson's paper the definite statement that one merely had to repeat the orders while allowing the manipulations to be made, together with several inferences, expressed above, I made from Alexander's aphorisms, gave me the information I had been looking for. The details in the training that provoked this frustration were:

A. The word "direct", in "direct your head upwards and forwards". It had, and still has, no meaning for me. The only alternatives I can think of as meanings for it are (i) say the words (ii) say the words and "wish" or "will" your head to go up and (iii) move it up. The word "direct" made me feel that there was some additional possibility that I could not grasp. I see no point in using this word at a time when it can have no content for the pupil. I suggest that something like "Give the order for the head to go forward and up", with the explanation that the pupil is to allow his body to be manipulated passively and then hold the position when the instructor lets go, would avoid this.

B. "Don't do anything"; "You are doing something". "Do something" to me means keeping some muscle tense. Doing nothing means letting them go slack. If one did this one would fall down if standing up, and even on the couch one's head would return to its former position as soon as the instructor let go of it. This clearly wasn't intended, and I found it frustrating not to know what it was I wasn't to do. If it were explained to the pupil beforehand that he should allow the instructor to make all the alterations, but retain the positions into which he is put, this would be avoided. I suggest too that instead of the ambiguous word "do", which has quite different meanings inside and outside of the Alexander Technique, one might say "Don't help me".

C. I wonder whether this practice in inhibiting responses might not be improved. As I've suggested above, it might be the most valuable part of the training. Instead of leaving the pupil to see the general possibilities of it himself, and to experiment on his own (apart from the "postural" stimuli), it might be valuable to subject him to other kinds of stimuli, giving him practice in inhibiting his reactions. This might be most effective if a series of stimuli were used which had more and more strong "emotional" tone for the pupil. One could find out the kind of situation, or behaviour in others, that brought about a particularly intense and uncontrollable habitual response, and then enact it for him to practise on. This would be well suited to work in groups. This is just a suggestion I have not thought about much yet. Perhaps you do something like this already. There is, however, one practical suggestion I would make. The first command, to which one should make no response, and the second, to which one does, are given in the same form. Frequently I did not know what my response to a given command should be, and I feel that they should be differentiated in some way.

THIRTY-FIVE

The South African Legal Action

A SUPREME COURT APPEAL at the end of 1949 marked the close of a legal action which was to be of the greatest importance to those engaged in education, physical education and medicine. Expert opinions were given by eminent scientists, including Sir Henry Dale, OM, FRS, Professor E. D. Adrian, OM, FRS, and Professor Samson Wright. The publications put into court as evidence covered a large field of physiology and medicine.

The general background to the legal action has been well summarized by Mr Norwood Coaker, KC (1949); but briefly the story is as follows. After some preliminary skirmishing, in and out of print, Dr E. Jokl, the physical-education officer of the South African government, published a strong attack in a government publication (1944) against the method of re-education described by F. M. Alexander. Dr Jokl's article was put forward as a scientific analysis of Alexander's method, but no scientist would have said that it was written in a scientific manner. In the words of the Appeal Judges of the Supreme Court: "It will be noticed that there is an appreciable quantum of malevolence in the article. It is not a dispassionate scientific analysis and consideration of the theories and claims in Alexander's books, but it directs ridicule and contempt not only at these theories and claims, but to some extent at the plaintiff in person."

The article was in fact couched in such terms that Alexander had little alternative but to request its withdrawal, and, when this was refused, to sue for defamation.

The case came up for trial in Johannesburg, before Mr Justice Clayden, in 1948. In the previous year evidence had been taken on commission at South Africa House in London from a number of scientists in this country. The South African government attorney undertook the defence of the editors of the publication, and Mr Oswald Pirow, KC, was briefed as counsel for defence. Judgement was given for Alexander in the sum of £1,000 with costs which ran into five figures, and this was confirmed in 1949 at the Supreme Court of Appeal, where it was found that the article was defamatory and not a fair representation of Alexander's theories.

The Alexander Method

In his brief summary of the Alexander method Mr Justice Clayden said:

The underlying concept is that man in early times was a creature whose bodily functions were regulated by instinct, instinct properly adapted to his needs in the course of evolution. With the rapid advance of civilization, instinctive control of the body has not kept pace with man's needs and has ceased to be a proper guide. The time has come for man to employ his intellect in the care of his body. Bad use of the body, when controlled by instinct, shows its effects in all human ills. How then is the body to be put under the control of the conscious mind?

The difficulty which has to be overcome is that "sensory appreciation" is defective. Misuse of the body is not realized. The wrong manner of use feels and seems to be right. To explain the way of misuse and to try to teach correct use in action fails, because as soon as man sets out to act he reverts to his instinctive way of action with its old misuse.

The first step then (in re-education) is to stop the existing habitual reaction to an impulse. Attention must be concentrated on the manner in which the body is to work, and then the proper manner of working will be ensured and the act to be done may be allowed to come about.

The relationship of the head to the neck and the neck to the back in activity, is held to be the chief factor in influencing the correct functioning of the body. Maintenance of the proper relationship at all times will ensure that all parts and organs of the body are working at their best. The mind is brought to bear on maintaining the proper relationship. That relationship, the "primary control", when maintained, will bring about the proper functioning of the rest of the body. By constant attention to the manner in which acts are performed, and especially constant attention to the head-neck-back relationship, the acquired manner of using the body will take the place of the wrong instinctive manner, and the body will function with the least effort and to the best advantage.

Terminology

Judge Clayden agreed that "in Alexander's book these ideas are tangled in a mass of words".

One of the chief difficulties in the whole action was to agree on a

K

terminology which would ensure that the witnesses were talking about the same thing. Judge Clayden early established the terminology which he would employ:

> Mainly the evidence relates to the effect of good body mechanics on health and the prevention of disease, and to the possibility that "alteration in posture," or the "better use" of Mr Alexander, can improve body mechanics. When I use the term "body mechanics," I shall use it as defined by Dr Goldthwait: "The mechanics of the function of all the parts of the human body—bones, joints, muscles, viscera and nerves." "Posture," I think, means the carriage of the limbs and body as a whole. Where in my view the question or the answer in evidence uses these words in some different sense, I shall mention it. Mr Alexander and Dr Barlow shun the word posture: to avoid confusion, I shall use for the technique of Mr Alexander the phrase "Proper Use".

Judge Clayden held that Mr Alexander's main principles were:

> that man's health is deteriorating: that a main reason for this is the misuse of the body: that the misuse of the body cannot be corrected (by ordinary methods) because of faulty sensory appreciation: that "proper use" can however be taught (by his method): that the maintenance of a proper head-neck relationship will to a large extent bring about "proper use": that "proper use," so taught, will improve health and prevent disease.... Whether misuse of the body may be a cause of deterioration in health is so bound up with the question whether the Alexander technique can improve health and prevent disease that it has to be considered with those matters.

These principles would, Judge Clayden suggested, have to be proved unsound if the defendants were to maintain their allegation that Mr Alexander's system "is quackery in the fields of physical education and medicine".

Influence of Body Mechanics on Health
Considering in detail the evidence whether good body mechanics cannot improve health and prevent disease, and whether "proper use" (the Alexander Technique) cannot bring about good body mechanics, Judge Clayden pointed out that

> Professor Samson Wright is only prepared to concede that posture could have bad effects in cases of grave abnormality. Professor

Adrian says that posture could obviously have bad effects, though he is not prepared to say what degree of abnormal posture would have those effects. He says that it is a commonly accepted view that good bodily functioning makes people less prone to disease. Sir Henry Dale says that "such use of the body as a whole as keeps it in good health" may affect certain diseases.

Dr Barlow in his evidence refers to various American authorities. Dr K. G. Hansson [1945], a doctor acknowledged by Dr Jokl to be an authority, . . . reaches the following conclusion: "The relation between health and body mechanics is soundly based on physical laws and on physiology. There is increasingly strong clinical evidence of posture and health being the cause and effect in many conditions." The book *Essentials of Body Mechanics* in *Health and Disease*, of which the chief author is Dr Goldthwait, also an acknowledged expert, has passages which have been referred to in evidence on the effect of good body mechanics in health and in the prevention of disease. In the preface, pp. V–VI, this is the view expressed: "the proper training of the body for the greatest physical efficiency and the early recognition and treatment of faults which lead to disease are the chief business of the physician. In this prophylactic rôle of medicine, the development of good body mechanics plays an important part." Dr Barlow also relies in support of his view upon *Principles and Practice of Physical Therapy*, edited by Professor Pemberton, and on the American Medical Association's *Handbook of Physical Therapy*, especially the passage at p. 118, reading "Clinical evidence strongly suggests an intimate relationship between body mechanics and health".

These books by recognized authorities, or published with sanction of a recognized body, can only be used in support of the evidence of Dr Barlow. But the effect of all this evidence, and particularly the statement of Professor Adrian that it is a commonly accepted view that good bodily functioning makes people less prone to disease is that it certainly cannot be said that the defendants have proved that good body mechanics cannot lead to improvement in health and in a general sense to the prevention of disease.

The Head-Neck Relationship
The next stage in Judge Clayden's judgment dealt in detail with the relationship of the physiological researches of the late Professor Magnus to the Alexander method. This arose out of the following inaccurate statement by Jokl (1944):

The cornerstone of Alexander's "conscious control" theories is a discovery allegedly made by the late Professor Rudolph Magnus, who is said to have established the existence of "the primary control of the individual". This legendary "primary control," we are told, if properly brought into play, enables man to subject not only all his muscular actions but also the work of his internal organs to the supervision of his will.

Judge Clayden ruled quite definitely that Alexander made no claim to be able to teach people to control the working of their internal organs. He pointed out that the only claims to "control" which Alexander made, came in passages of which the following is an example: "For example, though it is not possible to control the viscera directly, we can control directly the muscles of the abdominal wall which enclose the viscera." The manner in which Alexander links up "conscious control" with what he terms "the primary control", appears in the following passage from his writings:

Readers of my book, *The Use of the Self*, will remember that when I was experimenting with various ways of using myself in the attempt to improve the functioning of my vocal organs, I discovered that a certain use of the head in relation to the neck, and of the neck in relation to the torso and the other parts of the organism, if consciously and continuously employed, ensures, as was shown in my case, the establishment of a manner of use of the self as a whole which provides the best conditions for raising the standards of functioning of the various mechanisms, organs, and systems. I found that in practice this use of the parts, beginning with the use of the head in relation to the neck, constituted a primary control of the mechanisms as a whole, and that when I interfered with the employment of the primary control of my manner of use, this was always associated with a lowering of the standard of my general functioning. This brought me to realize that I had found a way by which we can judge whether the influence of our manner of use is affecting our general functioning adversely or otherwise, the criterion being whether or not this manner of use is interfering with the correct employment of the primary control. . . . This "primary control", called by the late Professor Magnus the "central control", depends on a certain use of the head and neck in relation to the use of the rest of the body. (Alexander, 1932)

Professor Samson Wright dealt carefully with this point and established that what Alexander was referring to as his "primary control" has nothing whatever to do with Magnus's concept of the Zentralapparat which refers to centres in the brain-stem. Summing up on this point, the Appeal Judges said:

It requires an appreciable amount of anatomical and physiological knowledge to understand the experiments of Magnus, and a considerable knowledge of technical terms to understand the published description of the experiments. The expert witnesses called for the defence say that Alexander's knowledge of these subjects is very limited and some of them suggest that he never read any description of Magnus's experiments but was given a second-hand account of them which he did not understand. It is furthermore clear that before Magnus published the results of his experiments Alexander had already in his two earlier books attached great importance to the proper carriage of the head and neck. In the circumstances it is impossible to infer dishonesty rather than conceit and ignorance on the part of Alexander in relation to his claim to have anticipated Magnus in his discovery of a "central control". It seems to be not at all unlikely that he saw some resemblance between his theory about the head-neck relationship and Magnus's experiments, based upon some vague understanding of what he had been told about those experiments, and came to the conclusion that what he had found out about the position of the head and neck was a discovery similar to the one made by Magnus.

Judge Clayden went on to point out that even if Alexander had misinterpreted Magnus in this one respect, this did not upset his own theory about the head-neck relationship.

Much of the evidence of the expert witnesses was given on the basis that Mr Alexander said that there was some centre in the body through which the mind could control the functions of the body. To show that Professor Magnus talked of nothing of the sort does not assist the defendants: such evidence proves only that what is not a basis of the Alexander technique is not sound. When asked instead to assume that all that the "primary control" meant was a relationship of the head to the neck, Sir Henry Dale, the intimate friend of Professor Magnus, says: "Magnus showed that the relation of the head to the neck has great reflex effects on all other parts of the body of the animal," and agrees that Magnus put forward the phrase "When the head moves, the body follows." Professor Adrian says the same. He says that what Magnus showed in animals "has not been shown in man," and gives as a reason the fact that in four-footed animals "the head is in a different relation to the body than it is in man". A passage from the book of Sir Charles Sherrington, *The Endeavour of Jean Fernel*, which reads "To take a step is an affair not of this or that limb solely but of the total neuro-muscular activity of the moment—not least of the head and neck," was a passage with which he agreed.*

Professor Samson Wright discussing the movement of the head in the normal actions says: "That would have effects on certain muscles in other parts of the body," and says it is "extremely difficult to demonstrate any significant change in organs other than the muscles" by reason of the relation of the head to the neck. Dr Jokl says that there might be a connection between what Professor Magnus showed in decerebrate animals and a changed posture in human beings by reason of a certain head-neck relationship, assuming that posture was so changed, but he says he would require proof of that connection.

In the world of science it is no doubt necessary for Mr Alexander to show that the maintenance of a certain head-neck relationship can in man improve the functioning of the body. In this case it is not necessary for him to do so. The defendants in their article have chosen to assert the contrary, and in this court have undertaken to prove that what they say is true. Challenges by witnesses to Mr Alexander to substantiate what he claims cannot prove the truth of what the defendants assert. Assuming that Mr Alexander can derive no support for his theory, that the maintenance of a certain head-neck relationship can have effects on the bodily functioning of man, from the works of Professor Magnus, because those works did not deal with man, still the defendants have to prove Mr Alexander wrong. It is a criticism then that he may wrongly claim support from those works, but the proof that he is wrong has to be given otherwise.

Does the Alexander Method Improve Body Mechanics?
Judge Clayden continued:

What has to be proved is that "proper use" (the Alexander method) cannot bring about good body mechanics. Professor Samson

---

* The sentence immediately preceding this in Sir Charles Sherrington's book reads "Mr Alexander has done a service to the subject by insistently treating each act as involving the whole integrated individual, the whole psycho-physical man."

Wright explains that a great many of the physiological reasons which Mr Alexander sets out in support of his technique are wrong. In his study of the technique which was only from the books, he has restricted himself entirely to Mr Alexander's physiology. . . . Very little of this evidence relates to the possibility of Mr Alexander's "proper use" bringing about good body mechanics. When witnesses do speak of posture, or the head-neck relationship, they seem to be referring to some pose which is adopted for a while for a particular purpose, and not to the maintenance of a position of advantage to the body in all activity of the body. The emphasis which was placed by Dr Jokl on the supposed "primary conscious control," and the alleged ability to control all organs, has I think caused the evidence to be mainly directed to showing how false such conceptions are. The evidence for the defendants . . . is designed rather to support Dr Jokl's article than to deal with the effects of Mr Alexander's technique in practice. In my findings on this part of the case I am not, I think, disregarding the very expert evidence which the defendants have led. The evidence could no doubt have discussed fully how far the Alexander Technique, as applied in practice, could lead to good body mechanics. But through the misunderstanding of the technique expressed in the article, it has not on the whole been led in this regard.

Dr Jokl, who gave evidence after the technique had been fully explained by the witnesses for the plaintiff, deals more directly with this matter. He denies that improvement in *posture* can bring about good body mechanics, but the grounds of the denial are, I consider, that improvement in posture brings about nothing, because it itself must be brought about by other factors, which are the factors responsible for improving the body mechanics.

As against this evidence there is the evidence of Dr Barlow. In the field of medicine he does not pretend to speak with the authority of the English witnesses, or Dr Jokl. What he does maintain is that he, as a doctor, has studied the Alexander Technique, and that he can therefore express with reason his views on the effects of it.

It is here that the defendants find themselves in a difficulty. What has to be proved is that the technique cannot improve health and prevent the diseases which it claims to prevent. . . . All of the witnesses for the defendants say that they cannot discover what Mr Alexander does to bring about "proper use," from his books: none of them has seen the technique in operation. . . . The defendants have in my view to prove not only that the system as described is unsound but that as described and in operation it is unsound. They have to prove, on the issue which I am now considering, that persons who have undergone a course of instruction from Mr Alexander or his teachers, do not thereafter have improved body mechanics. Since none of the defendants' witnesses have seen such a person this is difficult. The evidence which is given as to the absence of effects of altered posture is not, I consider, evidence which can show this, because the posture which is spoken of is not "proper use": it is not a position of advantage continuously maintained in movement. And the defendants do not offer proof that Mr Alexander's teaching does not in fact bring about improvement in body mechanics, whilst the plaintiff does offer such proof.

Judgment on the Soundness of the Method

In the absence of evidence showing on the balance of probability that "proper use", as taught, cannot improve body mechanics, and by reason of the evidence as to the effect of good body mechanics, the defendants have in my view failed to establish that the system is unsound. They have shown that Mr Alexander supports his technique by wrong physiological reasoning and by reference to work which almost certainly has nothing to do with it. But that in my view is not enough.

In regard to the claims to prevent disease, the defendants in the article said that a claim was made to prevent practically every known disease. This was not, I think, claimed in the books. In regard to the diseases which he does claim to prevent, although I am far from saying that the evidence shows that claim to be sound, yet I consider that the defendants have not proved the negative they had to prove: they have not shown that what might lead to improved health might not prevent diseases for which the causes, or factors which build up resistance, are unknown. They have failed in my view to prove that the system cannot bring about the results which it does claim in the improvement of health and the prevention of disease, and again they have made matters worse by overstating the claims made for the system. The claim to improve health has not been shown to be baseless, even in the medical field.

THIRTY-SIX

What Sort of Alexander Teacher?
by Dr Wilfred Barlow

IN MY BOOK, *The Alexander Principle*, I made the point that Alexander had not been too well served by some of his earlier supporters, but that an increasing number of younger teachers, who were now being trained in various centres, might be expected to serve him better. I fear though that I may have spoken too soon— far from the hoped-for development having taken place, there seems to be an increasing attrition of Alexander's ideas in some quarters, and some bizarre procedures are being passed off as the genuine article. Some of them bear little relationship to the Alexander Technique—for example, the following recent description from America:

> The technique begins with gentle exploratory manipulations of the neck muscles by the instructor, and gradually comes to involve the muscles of the entire body in a series of corrective adjustments. To discover the head-neck relationship necessary for optimal physical function, the practitioners of the technique advise the student to place the medial forefingers on the inferior occipital portion of his own head, with the thumb resting lightly on the anterior lateral portion of the neck, below the angle of the mandible. With training the student should be able to recognize postural errors and then learn to correct them.

The crudity and silliness of such a procedure would be apparent to anyone who had had genuine Alexander lessons.

The main attrition of Alexander's ideas, however, comes from the discarding by teachers of the basic Alexander concepts of "inhibition" and "direction". Accounts nowadays flood in of teachers who conduct their manipulative sessions in almost total silence, refusing to give any explanation beyond the manipulative experience: of teachers who combine their Alexander work with forms of dance or exercise, all of it to the exclusion of the "psycho" part of this psychophysical technique. One teacher wrote recently, "I am strongly opposed to pupils practising the given directions without the aid of the teacher's hands because it is my observation that they tense their necks, narrow their attention to one area and put themselves into fixation." Instead he gives his students "movements to practise". Since the essence of Alexander's work was what he called "directing", to be given "movements to practise" is about as far away from his work as it is possible to imagine. These and many other strange developments are very disquieting, and it may not be easy, if you are new to Alexander, to know whether you have got hold of a good teacher or not, though this does not mean, of course, that the majority of teachers are not excellent.

As in everything else, personal impressions are important, and a teacher who is right for one person may not be right for another. If a given teacher strikes you as odd after a few sessions, there is no reason to distrust your judgement—there is nothing about Alexander's work which should produce oddities, least of all in its teachers. There are of course temperamental factors in finding the right teacher—in the group of twelve who work at the Alexander Institute, we all recognize that some of us are better, say, with children or adolescents, some better with musicans, some particularly good with breathing problems; and so on, although all will give a sound basis of instruction.

The Alexander Story

Embarking on a course of instruction is for most people a totally novel and exciting adventure in which they begin to explore a quite new approach to their life. All of us, at any given time, are engaged in an evolving personal life story—the whole preceding history of our life as it carries on into the next new development. The development of the Alexander part of our "story-line" might seem to be arbitrary, depending upon which particular teacher we happen to have gone to. This should not be so, provided that the teacher's skill is adequate: the "plot" can only go in a certain direction, after the whittling away of misuses: the teacher has to help us find our way to it. But Alexander teachers do vary in their skill and experience: and whilst the initial excitement of the Alexander procedure may sustain interest for quite a long time, the pupil may become stuck because one particular teacher cannot help the development of the basic "plot". Everyone may get stuck at one point or another, whoever they go to, but the on-going sense of development should not be lost for more than short periods. This does not mean that the developing Alexander story is bound to be difficult and complicated—the Alexander influence may only be a small but vital part of a story-already-evolving. If well-given lessons do produce tension or mystification, it has to be the inevitable consequence for that particular person and not simply what is always likely to happen to everyone. Many "stories" develop without any mystification. However, if a teacher is inadequate, too much mystification may appear—important questions will be ignored, because the teacher's explanatory framework is not yet adequate.

Training Alexander Teachers

Why then should Alexander teachers—or any teachers for that matter —vary so much in quality or competence? After seeing the development of many teachers' stories over the years, there seems to be a series of stages in achieving maturity as a teacher. The first stage will have been one of *acceptance* of the need to have personal Alexander lessons. The next stage will be one of *choosing* to become an Alexander teacher and of joining a teacher-training group. It is often not until quite well on into the training that the third stage appears—one of clear *commitment* to make Alexander teaching the main career and mode of earning a living. This is a commitment which will often last a few years after finishing the actual training, but often in this stage there will still be other competing lines of development—an attachment to some other career and way of earning a living. This will be the stage at which the newly-trained teacher is still very excited by the Alexander ideas, but may no longer accept passively the values which his teachers have passed on. He may begin, in this stage, to attempt to shape the technique to fit in with other skills—an athlete may seek to combine it, say, with running, a musician with piano, voice or violin techniques, a dancer with various movement disciplines or yoga; a naturopath-lover perhaps with various other fringe activities: a devotee of esoteric disciplines such as Gurdjieff or meditation may begin to include some of these modes of "work" and "contemplation" in his Alexander instruction: and so on. Such an experimental phase may be an important one for many teachers, but likewise it may prevent full professional development into the next stage. I would of course include in this stage my own early medical assays.

The next stage is the important one and here the "amateur" phase begins to be left behind. Any previous experimental mixing of Alexander teaching with other forms of teaching is replaced by one of complete dedication to the Alexander Principle—the teacher's life becomes so constituted that the Alexander work is central to it, and no plan for living would be made which would seem likely to destroy this centrality. This fourth stage goes on into a fifth stage where there will be almost complete internal consistency of values—years of teaching experience will have ironed out most of the inconsistencies, and the alternative skills of stage three will have been so impregnated with the Alexander approach that both they and the mainstream of Alexander teaching will be advanced. At this high level of teaching maturity, there will probably be an ability to conceptualize values so that the teacher will keep on realizing that he is organizing his teaching in a more subtle and comprehensive way.

The last two stages—dedication and internal consistency—seem to me to be an essential requisite for a teacher who is going to train other Alexander teachers, and, ideally, for any Alexander teacher who is not teaching under the supervision of more experienced teachers. It is disastrous if teachers who are still at stage three should undertake the training of other teachers, however good their psychomotor skills may be. Indeed crude motor skills in handling people are not really too difficult to acquire, and these crude skills will fairly soon enable young teachers to alter their pupils' manner-of-use. But genuine Alexander teaching skill is a sophisticated combination of the psychological with the physical, and this takes a long time to mature.

It may be thought that I am seeking too much from Alexander teachers, and that we should be content with the instructive experiences which one person can give another manually without too much overlay of knowledge. Many might agree with one of my patients—an articulate if not literate mechanic—who listened patiently whilst I gave him what I thought were some real pearls of wisdom, and who then replied, "I see, if you stiffen your neck, you bugger the lot."

There are some Alexander teachers and pupils who regard this as a simple and beautiful truth and who think that this is "All ye need to know". Be that as it may, I take the view that teachers need to know a great deal more than the simple motor skills of manipulating: and that if all the pupil seems to be getting is the experience of being manipulated, then either the instruction is inadequate or else the pupil has not understood the rôle of "directing" both during the lesson and on his own.

Perhaps Alexander should have the last word: "You come to learn to inhibit and to direct your activity. You learn first to inhibit the habitual reaction to certain classes of stimuli, and second to direct yourself consciously in such a way as to affect certain muscular pulls."

List of Works Consulted

This list is not intended to be an extensive bibliography of writings on Alexander, but refers only to papers and other works mentioned in the text. Some are of considerable antiquity, including a few from the eighteenth and nineteenth centuries, but this is unavoidable when placing his work in its historical context.

Ashby, W. Ross (1952). *Design for a Brain*. London; Chapman and Hall.

Bach, C. P. E. (1759). Versuch über die wahre Art das Clavier zu spielen. Berlin.

Baines, Anthony (1976). *Brass Instruments, their History and Development*. London.

Barlow, W. (1947). Brit. J. Phys. Med. N.S., 10, 81.

—— (1952). Ann. Phys. Med., 1, No. 3.

—— (1954). Ann. Phys. Med., 2, No. 4.

—— (1956). Proc. Roy. Soc. Med., 49, No. 9, 670.

—— (1959). Brit. J. Clinical Practice, vol. 13, No. 5.

—— (1973). *The Alexander Principle*. London. Gollancz.

Behnke, Emil and Browne, Lennox (1887). *Voice, Speech and Song*. London.

Bell, Sir Charles (1852). Bridgewater Treatises, No. 4, 5th edition.

Booth, G. (1937). J. Nerv. Ment. Dis., 85, 637.

Bull, N. (1951). *The Attitude Theory of Emotion*. New York.

Cameron, N. (1947). *The Psychology of Behaviour Disorders*. Cambridge, Mass. USA. Houghton, Mifflin, Co.

Cannon, W. (1932). *The Wisdom of the Body*. London; Norton.

Coaker, N. (1949). Commerial Law Reporter. November.

Coates, Eric (1953). Suite in Four Movements. London.

Connolly, C. (1945). *The Unquiet Grave*. London; Hamish Hamilton.

Coster, G. (1934). *Yoga and Western Psychology*. London; Oxford University Press.

Covalt, D. A. (1949). Arch. Phys. Med., 30, 706.

Critchley, M. (1950). The Body Image. Lancet, 1, 335.

Culbertson, James T. (1950). *Consciousness, and Behaviour*. Iowa; Wm. C. Brown Co.

Dart, R. (1947). *The Attainment of Poise*. S. Afr. med. J., 21, 74.

Darwin, Charles (1872). *The Expression of the Emotions*. London; Thinkers Library Edition, Watts, 1945.

Dewey, J. (1928). Bull. N.Y. Acad. Med., 4, 3.

Dunbar, Flanders (1945). *Psychosomatic Diagnosis.* New York; Hoeber. London; Hamish Hamilton.

Duport, J. L. (*c.* 1806). Essaie sur le doigté du violoncelle à la conduite de l'archet. Paris.

Elliot, D. (1944). Ann. Rheum. Dis., 4, 22.

Ellman, P. (1942). Ann. Rheum. Dis., 1, 50.

Farmer, Henry (1904). *History of the Royal Artillery Band.* London.

Fink, D. H. (1945). *Relief from Nervous Tension.* London; Allen & Unwin.

Forrester-Brown, M. F. (1926). Brit, Med. J., 1, 690.

Fox, M. (1945). J. nerv. ment. Dis., 102, 154.

Garmany, G. (1953). *Muscle Relaxation as an Aid to Psychotherapy,* London; Actinic Press.

Gideon, S. (1948). *Mechanization takes Command.* Oxford; University Press.

Goldthwait, J. E. (1915). Boston Med. Surg. J., 172, 881.

Gregg, A. (1944). Brit. Med. J., 1, 551.

Halliday, J. L. (1937). Brit. Med. J., i, 213.

Hansson, K. G. (1945). J. Amer. med. Ass., 128, 947.

Havás, Kato (1961). *A New Approach to Violin Playing.* London.

Head, H. (1920). *Studies in Neurology.* London; Oxford University Press.

Hebb, D. O. (1949). *The Organization of Behaviour.* New York; Wiley.

Hench, P. (1946). Ann. Rheum. Dis., 5, 106.

Henley, E. (1932). Arch. Neurol. Psychiat. Chicago; 28, 629.

Herrick, J. (1948). *George Ellett Coghill.* Chicago; University of Chicago Press.

Hodgson, Percival (1934). *Motion Study in Violin Playing.* London.

Hooton E. (1936). Science, 83, 271.

Inman, V. (1952). Electroenceph. clin. Neurophysiol., 4, 192.

Jacobson, E. (1920). N.Y. med. J., 111, 419.

James, W. (1915). Gospel of Relaxation. In *Selected Papers on Philosophy.* London; Dent (Everyman Edition).

Johnson, W. (1946). *People in Quandaries.* London; Harper.

Jokl, E. (1944). Manpower, 2, 2.

Jones, E. (1957). *Sigmund Freud: Life and Work,* vol. 3. London; Hogarth.

Kay, Elster (1963). *Bel Canto.* London.

Keith, A. (1923). Brit. med. J., 1, 451.

Konorski, J. (1949). Mechanisms of Learning. In *Psychological Mechanisms in Animal Behaviour.* London; Cambridge University Press.

Kortland, W. (1940). Arch. névrl. Zool. 4, 401–520.

Kretschmer, E. (1951). Psychosomatic Medicine in Psychotherapy. Proc. R. Soc. Med., 11, 965.

Laplace, L. B. and Nicholson, J. T. (1935). J. Amer. med. Ass., 107, 1009.

Lashley, K. (1949). In Search of the Engram. In *Psychological Mechanisms in Animal Behaviour*. London; Cambridge University Press.

Lorenz, K. (1950). *Psychological Mechanisms in Animal Behaviour*. London; Cambridge University Press.

MacCulloch, W. (1951). Why the Mind is in the Head. In *Cerebral Mechanisms in Behaviour*. London; Chapman & Hall.

Mackay, D. (1951). Brit. J. Phys. Sci., 11, No. 6.

Mackinnon, Lilias (1938). *Music by Heart*. London.

Magnus, R. (1925). Proc. Roy. Soc., p. 339.

—— (1926). Lancet, 2, 531.

Malmo, R. (1949). Psychosom. Med. 2, 9.

Matthay, Tobias (1902). *The Act of Touch*. London.

—— (1932). *The Visible and Invisible in Piano Technique*. London.

Merton, P. A. (1953). In "The Spinal Cord." London; Churchill.

—— (1954). J. Physiol., 114, 183–198.

Mitchell, S. W. (1901). Treatment by Rest, Seclusion, etc., in Relation to Psychotherapy: J. Amer. med. Ass., 50, 2033.

Mozart, Leopold (1756). Violinschule. Augsburg.

Pemberton, R. (1947). *Principles and Practice of Physical Therapy*.

Pieper, J. (1952). *Leisure, the Basis of Culture*. London; Faber.

Plutchik, R. (1954). J. Gen. Psychol., 50, 1.

Prosser, E. M. (1948). *Manual of Massage and Movements*. London.

Rathbone, J. (1936). *Residual Neuromuscular Hypertension*. New York; Columbia University Press.

Reich, W. (1949). *Character Analysis*. New York; Orgone Institute Press.

Richards, I. A. (1952). *Practical Criticism*. London; Routledge & Kegan Paul.

Sainsbury, P. J. and Gibson, J. (1954). J. Neurol. Neorosurg. Psychiat., 17, 3.

Salter, A. (1950). *What is Hypnosis?* London; Athenaeum Press.

Schilder, P. (1935). The Image and Appearance of the Human Body; Studies in the Constructive Energies of the Psyche. Psyche Monogram No. 4, London; Kegan Paul.

Schultz, J. H. (1952). Das Autogene Training (Konzentrative Siebstentspannung). Stuttgart; Thieme.

Sheldon, W. H. (1940). *Varieties of Human Physique.* New York; Harper.

Sherrington, C. (1937). *Man on his Nature.* Cambridge University Press.

—— (1946). *The Endeavour of Jean Fernel.* London and Cambridge; Cambridge University Press.

Shaw, G. B. (1937). Preface to *London Music in 1883–89.* London; Constable.

Skynner, R. (1958). D.P.M. Thesis. London.

Suzuki, S. (1969). *Nurtured by Love.* New York; Exposition-University.

Sweet, C. (1938). J. Amer. med. Ass., 110, 419.

Szigeti, J. (1970). *Szigeti on the Violin.* London; Cassell.

Tanner, J. M. and Dupertuis, C. W. (1950). Amer. J. Phys. Anthrop., N.S. 8, 27.

Tegner, W. (1955). In Copeman, *Textbook of Rheum. Disease.* London; E. & S. Livingstone Ltd.

Thorpe, W. H. (1950). "Concepts of Learning". In *Psychological Mechanisms in Animal Behaviour.* London; Cambridge University Press.

Valéry, P. (1951). Trans. D. Bussy. *Dance and the Soul.* London; Lehmann.

Vannini, V. (1924). Della Voce Umana. Florence.

Walshe, F. M. R. (1951). "The Hypothesis of Cybernetics". Brit. J. Phil. Sci., 11, 161.

Walter, W. G. (1953). *The Living Brain.* London; Duckworth.

Whone, H. (1972). *The Simplicity of Playing the Violin.* London; Gollancz.

Wiener, N. (1948). *Cybernetics.* New York. Wiley.

—— (1950). *The Human Use of Human Beings.* London; Eyre & Spottiswoode.

Wisdom, J. (1951). Brit. J. Phil. Sci., 11, No. 5.

Wittgenstein, L. (1953). *Philosophical Investigations.* Oxford; Blackwell.

Wolff, H. G. (1948). *Headache.* London; Oxford University Press.

le Vay, D. (1947). Lancet, 1, 125.

Barlow.

(s) Alexander, F. matthias.

(n) Posture.

X